Mastering the Art of

Dressing

Well

Simple Steps to Successful Style

By Gillian Armour CIP

First Printing, March 2010
10 9 8 7 6 5 4 3 2 1

ISBN 9781449954871

Printed in the United States of America

Set in Calibri

Images used with permission: Microsoft, Gillian Armour, istock and Image Works.

For my nieces Sophia, Wilhelmina, Kyra, Sylvia, Julia, Erin and Sydney.

Introduction

Welcome to *Mastering the Art of Dressing Well*.

Becoming a best dressed woman takes knowledge and effort. And, in this day and age, just being a good dresser may not be good enough. You should strive to be *best-dressed* because appearances are so vitally important to your success and self esteem. Mastering this art can take years of practice and effort. I know because I do this for a living. As an image consultant I see the gamut of appearances, from those who are trying to look good (some even getting it!), to those who don't try at all. At times I am taken aback by the lack of care people seem to have for their appearance. Some must not realize that how they look is proportionate to how they are treated by bosses, colleagues and clients, as well as friends and family. Others might realize it but just don't know what to do.

This guide was written to help you clue into building a fashionable, *best-dressed* look using simple steps and easy tools. The goal of *Mastering the Art of Dressing Well* is to take away the mystery, to teach you that you can be better dressed, in fact *best-dressed,* by following a few fashion rules.

After years of observation and personal and professional fashion experience, I have learned a few things about looking *best-dressed* chic and I am going to share this knowledge with you in this guide. Once you understand and work with the fashion rules in *Mastering the Art of Dressing Well,* being *best-dressed* can be one of the easiest, most fun and rewarding things you do. So let me share one of the biggest lessons right now. Being a *best-dressed* woman takes being comfortable in your skin and being confident with who you are. I will return to this lesson many times in this guide.

With *Mastering the Art of Dressing Well* I am sharing my world, giving you the benefit of my years of practice and effort in the fashion world. My goal is to inspire you to create your own *best-dressed* look, to feel comfortable and confident with your fashion choices and to have fun celebrating your creativity doing it. So let's get going - use these basic tools of dressing to interpret your signature chic look and gain confidence doing so. Enjoy. *Gillian Armour*

What do you tell yourself about yourself?
Is it positive?

KNOW WHO YOU ARE

We are not born with a fashion sense, nor, for that matter, with any clothes at all. But as the years go by we develop a manner of dressing that is uniquely our own. It may not be in perfect taste or follow the style of the day, but it is our signature imprint and how we show the world our personality.

For the great majority of us, dressing to please ourselves works most of the time. We like comfort, like oversized sweatshirts for instance, but when personal style collides with fashion rules (usually work imposed) confusion sets in. Most of us eventually realize that how we look has an enourmous effect on others' opinions of us. By the time we get to college, or are ready for that shining career, we are both acutely tuned in to the impact of our appearance and painfully aware of how little we know about optimizing that appearance.

It's at this stage in your life where a guide to dressing well comes in handy – though it is never too late at any age. And, the first steps toward knowing the fashion rules become about knowing who you are. If you're about comfort why settle for conservative? Or if you're deeply artistic, why dress like a banker? Therefore it's important to know who you are as a person so you can shape and refine your sense of self-image. You want to be a step ahead in life whenever possible; it helps to have an outer look to match your inner personality.

Take time to discover the many aspects of your personality and challenge yourself to be yourself with the image you present to the world. To find out more about who you are and what your style personality is, take the short test on the next page. It's just for fun and, who knows, you might learn a thing or two!

WHO ARE YOU?

These questions are meant to stimulate you to making decisions about your existing style personality.

1) What is the most comfortable thing I wear?

2) What one outfit that I wear makes me feel fantastic?

3) When I wear the color_____ people always say I look great.

4) I am most confident when I wear _____

 5) If I could change one thing about myself it would be:

6) My favorite color combination is (choose only three; ex: *pink, grey, black).*

7) Of the following *style personalities* pick the one that describes you the best:

Conservative	Smart	Practical	Classic	
Modern	Poised	Romantic	Vintage	Charming
Dramatic	Independent	Sexy	Artistic	Creative
Passionate	Elegant	Cultured	Classy	

(It is important to narrow your style personality down to just ONE of these adjectives. Even if you think you might be a combination of several, pick one that describes you the MOST)

8) Write a paragraph and describe how it feels to be this style personality.

9) Describe how your outer look (hairstyle, makeup, accessories and dress) reflects this style.

10) Is this the style personality you want to have for the rest of your life? Is it the one that makes you feel confident, beautiful and fully expressive of self?

11) If you answered 'yes' to both parts of number 10 then you are ready to claim your individual style and you KNOW YOU ARE. If you did not have a clear answer, then take the **Style Personality** questionnaire on page 51.

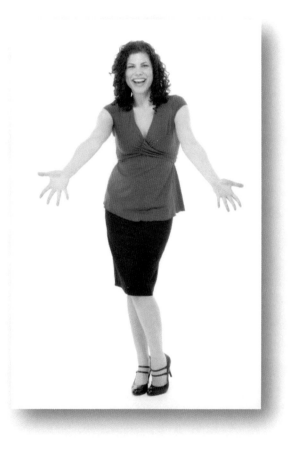

Know Your Personality?

Is your style personality congruent
with who you really are? Or, are
you trying to look like someone else?

KNOW YOUR COLORS

Every season designers introduce new colors in their new clothing lines. It is easy to be tempted to try some new colors for the new season. Don't do it unless these colors are right for you. The truth is not all colors look good on everyone. With every item you enter into your wardrobe, be sure its color will look good with your skin type and hair color so that you will always look the most flattering.

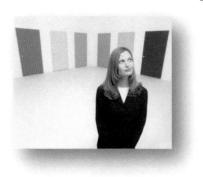

The best way to be sure what colors are best on you, and to be confident every time you get dressed, is to have your colors professionally assessed by a certified color consultant or other certified image professional. They will give you a color palette that you can take with you shopping, to match against new pieces that you are considering adding to your wardrobe. Here are a few tips and tricks to help you understand more about color:

Dispel Myths

There are some myths that just need to be tossed out the window. A good example is the common assumption that redheads should stay away from anything pink or red. The truth is that, depending on the strength of the red in the hair, it is quite possible for these women to use clothing with red in it. Take a second look at any coloring myths that you have heard and dare to buck them if you feel that you really do look good in these colors.

Take Time to Test

Take a selection of colors both warm and cool, light and dark, stand in front of the mirror in a well-lit room with natural light and hold each one up. Place it around half your face, chin and one side, to get an accurate idea. You will find that some colors tend to make you look pale or yellowish, 'washed-out' or otherwise just not 'nice'. These are the colors you should NOT be using in your wardrobe. The colors that make your cheeks glow, eyes sparkle and that go with your hair are the ones that should definitely be included.

Note Your Skin Tone

Everyone has an underlying skin tone. Some people have red or pink undertones, while others have yellow or blue. This undertone will have a major bearing on what colors look good on you. Usually if you pinch the skin on the back of your hand, the underlying color will be revealed for a few seconds. In general, people with blue or rosy undertones look best in winter colors like brown, white, navy blue and pastel colors. Pink or blue undertones with pale skin go best with cool summer tones like lavender, pink, blue, etc. Women with golden undertones do well with warm autumn colors; earth tones, grays and olives are all a good fit for this skin type. And 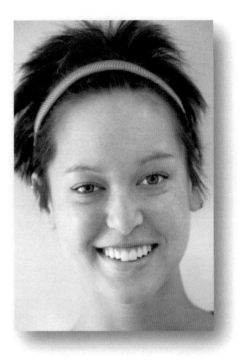 women who look good with spring colors like peach, bright blues and reds tend to have a very light skin with light golden undertones.

Use Buffer Colors

When you have a color that you like, but it does not particularly go with your skin tone, you can use a buffer color. Let's say you see a lovely black shirt that you like, but it washes you out and makes you look pale. Try picking one with a collar or add a scarf in a color that does look good on you to buffer the black from your skin. This can work with two pieces of clothing, as well. Put the color you love but does not look good on you on the bottom and a shirt that flatters you on top . . . the shirt acts as a buffer.

Knowing which colors look best on you is only the beginning. Now you need to make sure that your wardrobe is made up of these colors. Go through your closet and give away or donate everything that is in a color that doesn't work for you and then replace them with the correct colors. You'll be amazed at how much more flattering your outfits will be.

Tips to remember:

- Dare to buck color myths
- Always test colors next to your face
- Try matching base makeup to your skin
- Add accessories as buffers to flatter your skin tone
- Get a professional color analysis and save money by buying clothes that flatter your skin tone

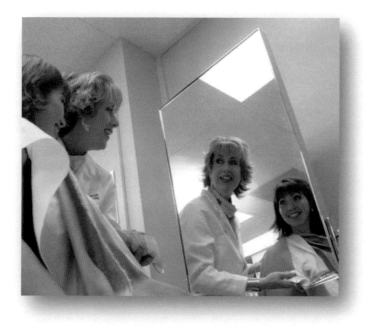

Professional Color Analysis

If you could choose just ONE color to represent who you are what would that color be?

DRESS FOR YOUR BODY TYPE

Most women realize that choosing clothes that are flattering to their body type is the best way to look great. If you do not pay attention to your body type, or don't know what it is, the result can be poorly assembled outfits that do not make you look your best.

The following tips will give you the knowledge necessary to choose the right clothing for you in particular. You will be able to dress easily in clothes that flatter your body type, rather than staring into your closet wondering what to wear.

What's My BodyShape / BodyStyle?

There are the five body shapes for women: the hourglass, triangle, inverted triangle, diamond and rectangle. Your body measurement determines which **one** of these you are. Everything you wear should harmonize with this defined body/shape in order to make you look your best.

- In order to flatter each body/shape there are "rules" of dressing.
- One has to understand line, proportion (or scale), silhouette and cut and how they relate to clothing your body/shape.
- Each body/shape is different and will look different in certain styles and sizes.
- Making your individual body/shape look fabulous takes a skillful combination of all of the above.

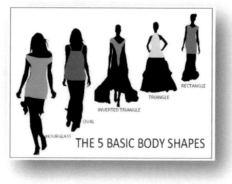

In these next few pages we will drill down with a series of charts for you to complete. Once measured you can determine your body shape (hourglass, oval, triangle, inverted triangle or rectangle) from the information below. Use the measurement charts on pages 105-109 to determine your unique shape.

_____BUST should be 8-10" larger than waist; if more, large bust; if less, small bust
_____WAIST should be 9-13" smaller than hips; if more, small waist; if less, large waist
_____HIPS should equal shoulder width; if wider, wide hips; if narrower, narrow hips
_____SHOULDERS from top of arm to top of arm across width of back
_____BACK LENGTH from base of neck to natural waistline in back
_____HIP WIDTH circumference from front of hips between waist and crotch
_____1) Top of Head to Floor (Your Height)
_____2) Bust to Floor
_____3) Hips to Floor
_____4) Mid-Knee to Floor

- The last four measurements will determine if your body is in proportion or not.
- If the measured inches between all four are even then you have a balanced body.
- If, for example, the distance between the top of your head to your bust is GREATER than the distance between hips to floor you are short legged.

Balanced Body   Short Legged   Long Legged

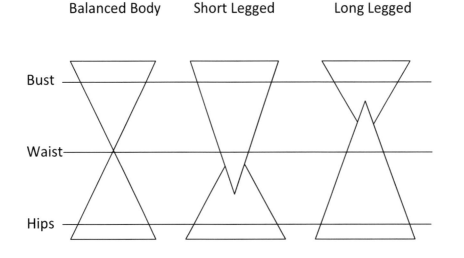

Bust

Waist

Hips

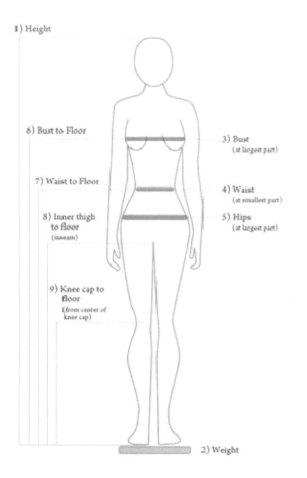

1) Height

6) Bust to Floor

7) Waist to Floor

8) Inner thigh
to floor
(inseam)

9) Knee cap to
floor
(from center of
knee cap)

3) Bust
(at largest part)

4) Waist
(at smallest part)

5) Hips
(at largest part)

2) Weight

Body Measurement	Inches
Height	
Weight	
Bust (At the fullest part)	
Waist (at the narrowest)	
Hips (at the largest part)	
Bust to floor	
Waist to floor	
Inner thigh to floor (inseam)	
Knee cap to floor	

To help you identify your shape we have listed the FIVE basic body shapes for women along with their identifying characteristics:

HOURGLASS

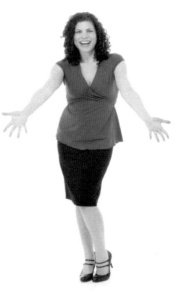

The ideal body shape and very easy to clothe.

Characterized by:

- Waist that is 9" to 13" smaller than the bust and hip measurements
- Bust and hips usually the same width
- Horizontal figure type versus vertical type (rectangle)
- Has waist definition
- Has a proportioned body
- Legs are in proportion but this body type may also have shorter legs

DIAMOND

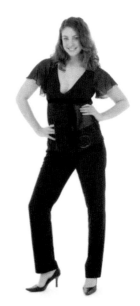

A very common body shape. The goal is to use clothing lines to create an hourglass shape.

Characterized by:

- Apple shape Fullness at midriff
- Smaller shoulders, sloping shoulders
- No waist definition
- Bust, waist and hips very close in measurements
- Usually has great legs but may have short legs combined with broad shoulders
- This body type also known as "oval" or "round"

RECTANGLE

This is also a very common body shape particularly for women over 50. At first glance this shape is boxy. The goal with this body type is to use clothing lines to create an hourglass shape by focusing attention on the waist itself. The proper use of color in clothes to camouflage works well with this shape.

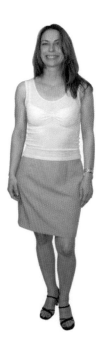

Characterized by:
- Very little or no waist definition
- Hips and shoulder width is balanced
- Small derriere
- Legs usually long
- Waist measures from 1" to 8" smaller than bust (if waist is more than 8" smaller this is an hourglass)
- This body type is also known as "column" or "square"

TRIANGLE

 A very common body shape as well. Many women tend to gather weight at the hips. The goal with this body type is to use clothing lines to create an hourglass shape.

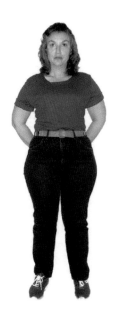

Characterized by:
- Small to medium size frame
- Narrow or sloping shoulders
- Hips wider than shoulder and bust line
- Body larger below the waist than above
- May have small bust line
- Full legs. Sometimes short legged, large hips and derriere
- This body type also known as "pear shaped"

INVERTED TRIANGLE

Often seen as an athletic shape because of broad shoulders. The goal with this body type is to use clothing lines to create an hourglass shape by focusing attention on the lower part of the body. Use clothing to make hips appear larger.

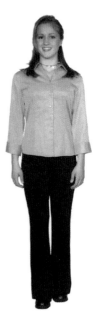

Characterized by:
- Shoulders wider than hips
- Body larger above the waist than below
- Small hips and a flat derriere
- May have a full bust, wide chest
- Great legs
- May have short legs combined with broad shoulders
- Waistline is not indented rather it is tapered to narrow hips

Now that you have identified your basic body shape you can feel confident choosing silhouettes that are the best for that shape.

If you are still uncertain about your particular body shape review the measurement charts on pages 105-109.

Bring Out Your Assets

No matter how many flaws you have, or think you have, you also have assets. The best way to look great is to downplay your body flaws and accentuate your assets. For example, if you have great legs, but are a little heavy in the hips, opt for a slender skirt in a darker color to minimize your hips and still show off your nice legs.

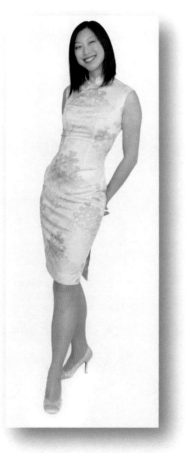

Likewise, if you have a good chest and a not so great stomach . . . use a plunging neckline to show off your asset and distract from your little bulge. Find ways to draw attention to your best parts and you'll find that you look and feel better.

Use Color to Change Shape

Your body is probably not perfect – not many are. But a little color goes a long way toward creating the look you want. Dark colors slim, while light colors tend to expand and bright colors draw attention. Use this to your advantage. If you have a pear-shaped body, with wide hips and a narrow top, try using dark-colored pants with a light top to balance things out. A bright scarf will draw attention away from the wider hips. This color principle will help you choose clothing to create the perfect look.

Find Flattering Cuts

When choosing pants, look for a cut that will enhance and balance your body type. A small waist and hips look great with tapered pant legs, while a large bottom can be slimmed by choosing a flared skirt or boot cut pants. Likewise, a crisscross or ruffled top will enhance a small chest by adding more bulk, while a plain shirt with only darts will look great on a larger chest. Peasant shirts, which are more flowing, flatter a smaller torso and fitted tops look better on larger women.

Use Accessories to Your Advantage

Accessories can be your best friend. Not only do they help distract from areas you don´t want people noticing, they can really add flair to your wardrobe and help you make your clothes look better on you. For example, if you are quite tall and want to look a little shorter, a wide belt can help create that illusion by providing a "cutting" line at your waist, which stops the eye. When the eye can move the length of the body without interruption, this creates the illusion of length, and so it stands to reason that a belt that creates an interruption would cause the body to appear shorter.

Knowing how to choose clothes that enhance your body type will result in a boost in your confidence. You will end up wearing outfits that look excellent on your body and leave you feeling great. The best way to get started is to use the above guidelines to get rid of any clothing that doesn´t suit your body type and then hit the stores to find something that does suit you. Once you have redesigned your wardrobe, there will be no more wondering which outfit will look right on you . . . everything will be just right.

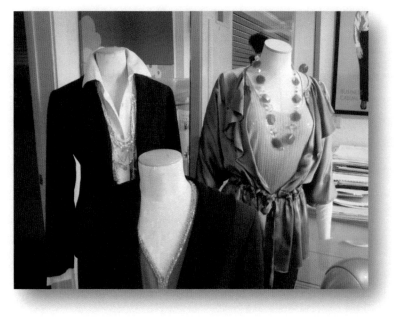

Accessories Add Flair to Your Wardrobe

ALL ABOUT FIT

Get The Perfect Fit

These days sizes on tags mean little since the actual sizes vary so much between designers and different clothing lines. Recognize that it does not matter how gorgeous or well-made a garment is, if it does not fit you properly it will not look good.

Unfortunately, most women do not know how important it is to get a good fit and as a result, they have a wardrobe full of pretty, yet unflattering clothing. The solution is quite simple: get clothes you buy to fit you properly. The following tips will provide you with the knowledge necessary to find clothes that fit and flatter your body, no matter what size you are. With the right clothing anyone can look stunning.

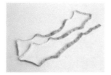 ## Find Out Your Real Measurements

Do not mentally rely on those measurements you took a few moments ago. Knowing your real size in inches is vital to getting a proper fit, so get out the tape measure and take those measurements again. Write them down so you´ll remember and be sure to check your measurements at least every six months so you can shop for the right fit.

Look for Width Before Length

If you are going to have to alter your clothing, it´s almost always easier to shorten than it is to change the width. So, when you are doing your shopping, make sure that the clothing you select fits around you properly even if it´s too long. For example, jeans that are a perfect fit in the hips and waist are almost always too long for most women. This can be altered and, in fact, many stores offer this service.

The part that matters in your pants is the waist and hips, since these are the areas that people will be noticing and, of course, it is also important to feel comfortable. For shirts, the shoulders and chest are the important parts. Even if the sleeves are too long, or the waist is too wide, this can be altered as long as the shoulders are in the correct position and you have no pulling in the chest area. The sleeve seam should hit the edge of the shoulder, as opposed to hanging down the arm or being too close to the neck.

Use the Right Foundation Garment

When you go shopping for new clothes, it´s important to wear the proper undergarment to try on clothes. Don´t use a tummy flattening panty if that is not what you would normally wear under your clothing. A good bra is essential, particularly if you are large-chested, since you will need to see precisely how tops hang when you are well supported.

Aim for Fitted, Not Skin-Tight

There is a saying – "skim, not skin" – that works well when you are choosing clothing for fit. Your clothes should not be like a second skin; they should fit close enough to look good, but not reveal every bump and lump on your body. On the other hand, baggy clothing is most definitely not flattering either, so try to get something between too loose and too tight. Just skimming the body is ideal.

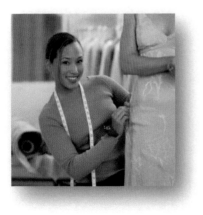

Find a Good Tailor

It is fine to drop off your pants at the dry cleaners if they need a hem, or if a shirt needs shortening at the sleeves. However for your jackets, suit pants, and outfits for dressier functions, find a good tailor. Ideally you want one with experience, someone who really knows how to modify a garment. Depending on your body shape, you may, for example, need to take the shoulders in on every jacket to get the best look; this is not an easy job so you want to have a tailor you are confident in to do this delicate work.

A Little More About Tailors and Seamstresses

A seamstress/alterationist is someone who can tailor (verb) (fit it to your body) and alter clothing, fix any damages to clothes and sometimes create custom designs. A tailor (noun) is someone who custom designs, creates and fits clothing for both men and women. Sometimes they do fixes but it is not their forté. A dry cleaner cleans clothes and sometimes fixes the holes, missing buttons, falling hems, and so on.

So decide what you need done by gathering that pile of fixables and sort into three piles. Pile one contains garments that are too big, too small, too short or too long. Pile two has items that are ripped, torn, have holes or are damaged in some way. Pile three just needs to be cleaned.

Next, pack pile number one up and head off to your local seamstresses for some quick fixing. When working with a seamstress, it's important to trust that they know how to pin and tuck to fit. Your job is to let them know during the pinning/fitting when you feel comfortable in your clothes. Their job is to adjust things to your liking and sew away. Expect to wait a few days to get your "new" clothes back. And remember to try on your items before you pay; if there are adjustments that were missed or that hem wound up way too short, you'll be able to leave that piece to be fixed again.

You'll also be taking pile two to the seamstress/alterationist or even dry cleaner to be mended. Again, expect to wait a few days for your items to be ready. Pile three, since all these items are is in need of the dry cleaner's care, goes to them. Soon you'll have a bunch of "new" clothes that are ready to impress. Because who wants to look at you in your ripped, dirty, ill-fitting garments?

Do An Assessment

This might be a good time to go through your closet and try anything on that you wear a lot or have not worn in a long time. Evaluate the fit, see if anything is ready to retire or if there are any alterations to be made. Knowing what pieces in your wardrobe need to be replaced, and/or what pieces you are missing, will help you use your shopping time most effectively.

Getting the proper fit is often more of an exercise in patience than anything else. When we buy something we want to wear it right away. Instead, wait until you have the proper fit. When your clothes fit great, you will feel and look great every time.

To help you edit and analyze your existing wardrobe we have provide worksheets (see pages later in this book) for you to pull out and use.

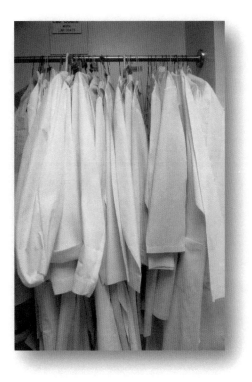

DRESS BASICS

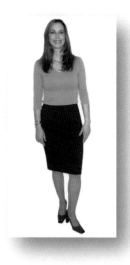

How you craft your individual style depends a lot of how comfortable you are with who you are. Be aware of your inate attractiveness and don't hesitate to offer it to the world. Just remember not to fall for the urge to overdo. Fashionable women learned this trick ages ago - restraint is the key to elegance. If you find that you want to add just one more piece to your outfit - don't.

Keep Your Budget in Mind

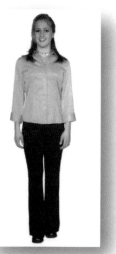

Once you put together your shopping list, do not just grab your purse and go. Do some Internet research to see what is out there, look for sales and calculate what a realistic wardrobe budget might be. You won't feel good in your new clothes if you have gone into too much debt for them.

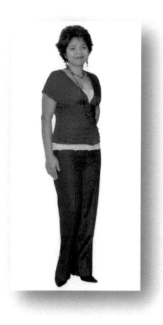

Invest in Quality

When shopping, remember that quality is important and you are going to spend more for quality. Leave trendy clothes for your weekend activities. Start with clothes that will last for at least a few years. Or, as we mention later in the book, shop your closet. You never know what new combinations you come up with until you've taken a fresh look at what you already own!

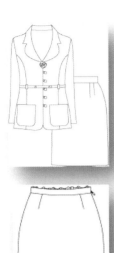

Essential pieces

While the task of getting your closet into "best-dressed shape" may seem daunting, this list will help you find the essential pieces to start with to build your wardrobe. Paste photos or draw illustrations of clothes from your closet in the spaces provided:

1.   Two dark suits in one of your core neutral colors (these are the colors that appear in your eyes and hair).

2.   One dark skirt in one of your core neutral colors.

3.   Two pairs of slacks in one of your core neutral colors.

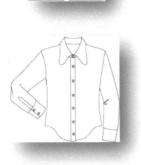

4.   Two solid shirts or blouses (not prints) in your accent colors.

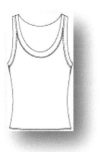

5.   Two accent-colored shells that would look great under your suit jackets.

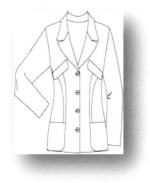

6.   A jacket that is tailored, yet loose, in an accent color.

7.   A knit shell in one of your core neutral colors.

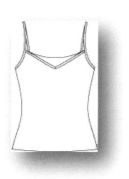

ADD YOUR ILLUSTRATIONS HERE:

Investment Dressing

How often have you thought you had found a great deal on a blouse or a dress and bought it on a whim, only to get home and discover that it practically disintegrated with the first washing? All too often, we are taken in by these so-called deals that are really just low prices for low quality clothing. It is a waste of money and time as well. Spending $200 a month on these poorly constructed clothes means you are wasting $2,400 a year!

Investment dressing requires you to pay more money per item of clothing, but you are going to be getting high quality items that will look and feel great and last a long time. The trick is to spot these smart buys that will help you build up an investment wardrobe that you can use for years to come.

Know Your Colors

Getting your colors done does not seem to be as much the rage as it has been in years past. This is a mistake. One of the smartest investments you can make to always look great and to not waste money when you shop is to get your colors professionally done so you feel confident a color will look good on you before you make a purchase.

Look for Timeless Pieces

There is something to be said for the little black dress that is appropriate for all occasions. If you look for clothing that has lines that aren't trendy, but always look good, no matter the latest style, you have a winner. This includes pencil skirts, sheath dresses and simple blouses. These are items of clothing that could hold their own in any decade, not for being at the height of fashion, but for their simplicity and quiet class.

Go for Quality Fabrics

Paying more for clothing that is made of better fabric is a smart decision. In fact, the type of fabric used in your clothes can make all the difference in how good you look. A cheap polyester dress will look far worse than the exact same design in a classy linen blend. Choose the better fabric and you won't regret it. Real silk, linen and wool are all fabrics that look terrific and will help build your investment wardrobe. Blends are fine too. Wool blends will be less itchy, linen blends will wrinkle less and silk blends will usually breathe more.

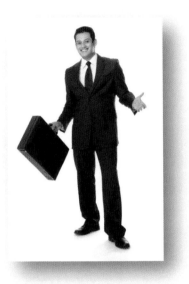

Remember That More is Not Better

Having a few expensive, classic pieces of clothing in your wardrobe is worth far more than having two or three closets full of cheap clothing that will never pass as good quality. Make sure you remember this when sticker shock hits!

If you have traveled to Europe, you have probably noticed how great the men and women look. They do not have as many clothes in their wardrobe yet most everything they have is made of the highest quality.

Make It All Work Together

The best way to build your investment wardrobe is to plan your entire wardrobe for versatility. Having two or three pairs of pants, three to five blouses, a couple of skirts and a nice jacket and suit can actually work for you if you plan it. Choose just two or three classic colors that all complement each other and you'll be able to mix and match your entire wardrobe, creating dozens of different outfits. Throw in a scarf or two and a couple of different belts and accessories and you can have even more looks, all with just a few select items. Opting for mostly solid colors rather than prints will give you more combinations as well.

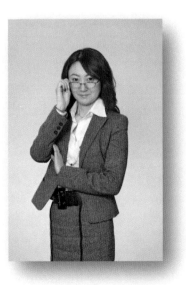

Remember the Shoes

Choosing the best shoes available will also enhance your look. Invest in a few pairs of good quality, sensible shoes and you will be able to wear them with every outfit. A couple of different high heels, a pair of flat shoes and perhaps some boots or sandals, depending on where you live, will serve you well and, when chosen in classic colors that suit your wardrobe, you'll never have any problems putting together a great outfit.

Investment dressing is becoming a trend these days and it's one that is well worth jumping on. Take a few minutes to plan out your basic wardrobe and choose a couple of colors to base it on. Then it's time to go shopping. Stick to the plan, choose high quality items; at the end of your day, you'll have a wardrobe that will last you a long time and suit any occasion.

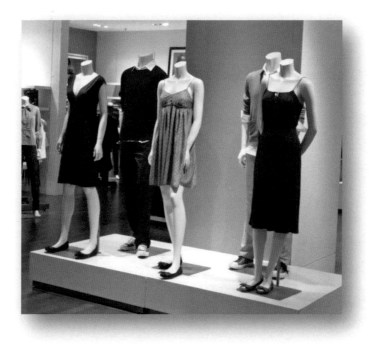

Plan Your Wardrobe Then Go Shopping

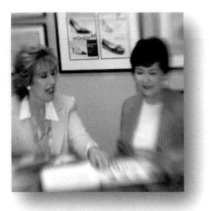

When In Doubt Hire a Professional

Consider hiring an image consultant, a personal branding coach, or an executive coach to work with you to define your professional objectives and help you put together your best possible executive wardrobe.

"I consulted Gilliam Armour in her capacity as a professional Image Consultant during the interval October, 2005, through February, 2006. The purpose of the consultations was to enhance my effectiveness in numerous public interactions including testifying in court. These public interactions are an important part of my job."

"Gillian developed a Personal Style Portfolio for me based on discussions of my objectives, a personality analysis, body type determination, color analysis, and subsequently at my home a wardrobe edit. We concluded the consultation by a shopping trip during which we expanded my wardrobe to include items which help me look and feel my very best."

"Gillian's work has greatly increased my confidence, and therefore my effectiveness, in my public interactions." *Dr. W. Satisfied Client*

To give you an idea of how to dress appropriately we've gathered a few of our favorite examples of well dressed men and women before and after their fashion makeovers.

Before and After

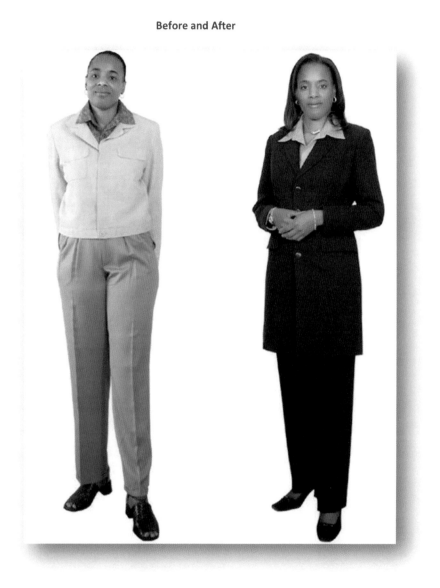

Good on the left and better on the right. "Before" she styled her clothing silhouettes inappropriately for her body shape. The boxy jacket made her look boxier and the duo-tone colors of her clothes created a horizontal line that visually chopped her in half!

Before and After

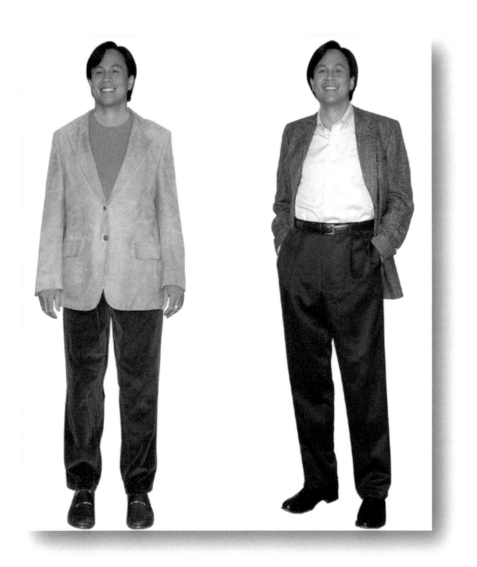

Sloppy fit and incorrect silhouette gave this gentleman a frumpy look (on left). With a fitted suit and pants that suit his body frame he looks much better.

Before and After

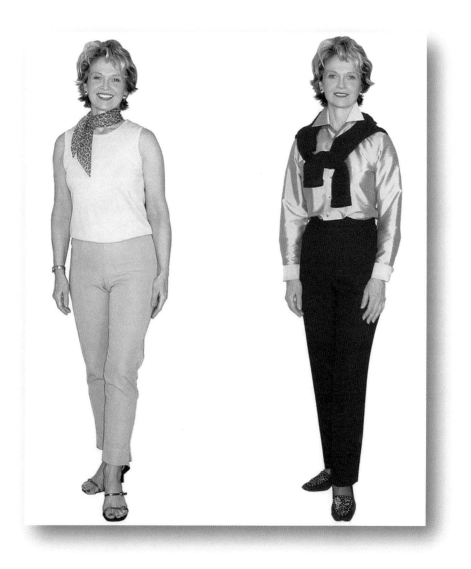

Age and style appropriate. When clothing fits too tightly on the body, the image sends many messages, amongst them - I don't care, I have let myself go, I don't respect you enough to dress well for you and I have bad taste. These messages may or may not be true for the wearer but for the viewer they are.

Before and After

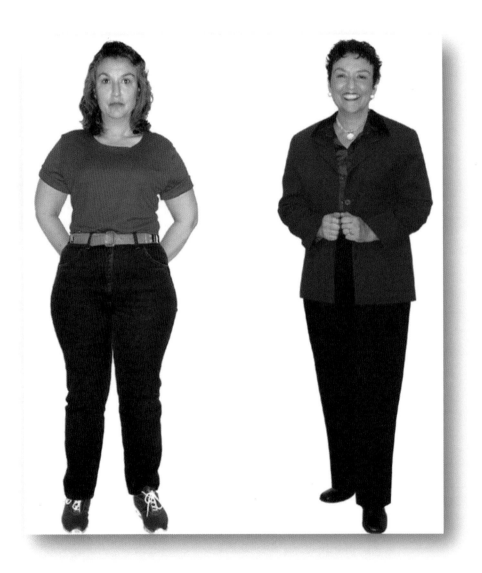

When you know your body shape and size you know how to clothe and camouflage it. The goal is always to flatter a woman's body with clothing and not to insult it as we see here (on left).

Before and After

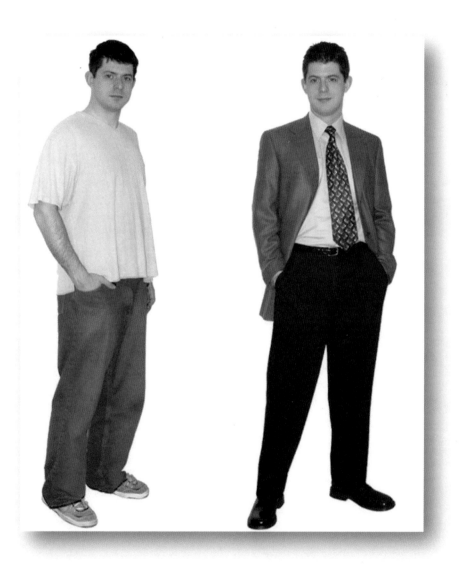

Business casual takes victims in the business environment. This young man might be the CEO of a technology firm but you'd never know it when he wears his jeans and t-shirts to work. With a suit and tie he gets the respect due him.

Before and After

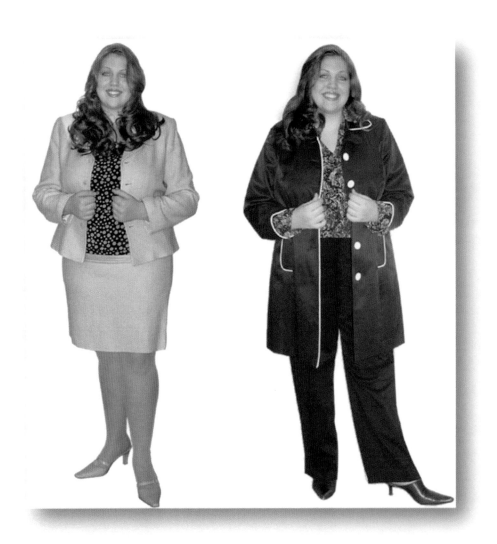

Plus-size figures can look great in clothes that are proportioned and that flatter. The goal is to camouflage problem areas and to wear clothing lines that slim and lengthen. Here the client chooses colors that minimize and heighten (on right).

Before and After

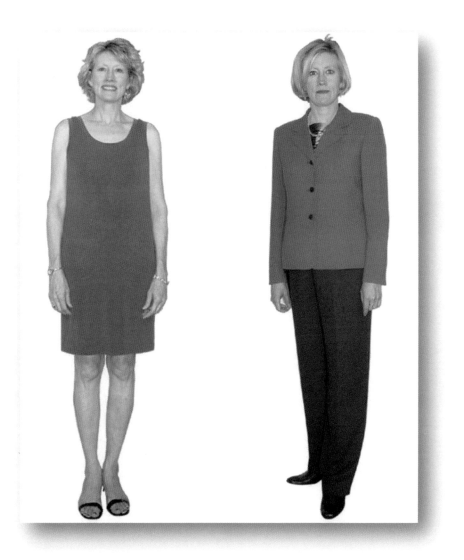

Be careful how you represent yourself to the world. If you are trying to convey a feeling of youth because you have reached a certain age, do it appropriately – with flattering clothes and gorgeous accessories.

Your Existing Wardrobe

Your budget tells you that you cannot afford another thing, and besides your closet is already full of great clothes to wear. So what if some are last year's styles? The phrase that defines the new shopping trend -"shop your closet" - is apropos for the economic climate we're in. Most of us are saving our pennies and not investing in new clothes. Our old shopping habits have died, hard. Now it's time to "make do with what you have." You can still wear your old clothes this year – all it takes is a little innovation and creativity to learn how to style these old looks into new ones! Re-fashion your existing wardrobe by looking at your clothing collection with newer, fresher eyes.

First, Study Current Trends to Get Ideas

One of the best resources for studying clothing trends is online at style.com. Here you get visuals, trend reports and exciting video. Use these guides to determine the trends you want to appropriate for yourself. Deciding which current looks you like helps you work with what you already own.

Next, "Shop" Your Closet

Remember when you used to shop by season? Spring would follow winter and that was the time to purchase lighter sweaters and pastel colors. Then summer would follow spring and you'd go buy a selection of shorts, dresses and hot weather tops, not to mention sandals and hats and sunglasses! So let's follow this concept and pay a visit to our closets.

Think about the season you are in right now. As I write, it's summer and 90 degrees outside. My goal for dressing on days like this is comfort and coolness. Heading to my closet, I'm looking for breezy tunics and oversized shirts to pair with leggings. I'll also be on the lookout for shirtdresses, or long t-shirts I can belt and slouch over shorts or Capri's.

But by themselves, these pieces can be run of the mill. I want to switch up my styling and get a newer, fresher look out of these "older" pieces. Check out current magazines or online fashion sites to see what's happening in fashion

NOW. When you see looks that appeal to you try to translate the looks by using what already exists in your closet. For instance, last year's peasant blouses can be transformed this year by tucking them INTO your jeans or skirts.

Here are a few more last year/this year suggestions:

- Last year's ombréd looks: layer them this year. Put a silk cami over last year's ombré tank top, then pair with mid knee leggings for a whole new look.
- Last year's oversize men's white shirt: add a colorful belt and an enormous/bold necklace. Wear over a pair of skinny jeans (also from last year).
- Last year's transparency trend – this year wear something over it.

You get the idea – develop your styling skills by reviewing last year's clothes and re-interpreting them into this season's hot looks.

Finally, much of fashion changes only slightly from one year to the next. Silhouettes are re-interpreted by designers to look fresh. Stylists take last year's looks and re-fashion them by tailoring or changing the cut of a jacket, pants or top to make them more relevant to today's trends. You can easily do this yourself.

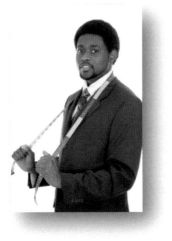

Find a good alterationist or tailor who can help you achieve your vision. Have an idea in mind for converting the item you have pulled from your closet. Jackets can easily convert to sleeveless vest styles. Skirts can be made longer or shorter depending on the mood of the fashion moment. Pants can be made into Capri's or shorts and even short-shorts if you are young enough to carry off the trend.

So don't let your limited imagination stop you from getting creative with your closet – trust me, the minute you start to look at your clothes in a new light your imagination will ignite and you will create hot new looks. You'll have tons of new things to wear!

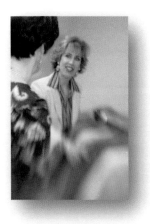

Wardrobe Edit Worksheets

To help you plan and manage your executive wardrobe I've included the following worksheets and planners. Use the following to go through your closet, identify items that no longer belong in your possession, and create new outfits to wear!

Step 1 CLOSET INVENTORY - make a list of everything in your closet and decide to keep, fix, tailor or donate.

Step 2 WARDROBE PLANNER - use this worksheet to create coordinated outfits from the edited clothing pile.

Step 3 FOUNDATION PLAN - for a nine piece coordinated set of clothing. With just 9 pieces from your wardrobe that match these silhouettes you can create 42 separate and matched outfits.

Step 4 OUTFIT PLANNER - gives you the option of creating Business Casual, Business Dressy, Business to Event or Event outfits.

Step 5 ACCESSORY WORKSHEET - use this worksheet to coordinate jewels, hats, purses, shoes, etc with your outfits.

> Letting go of favorite clothing items
> is emotional. To soften this experience
> when editing your closet, spend time with the
> memories of your special pieces. Then wish them goodbye and
> perhaps donate them to a favorite cause or charity.

Step 1

CLOSET INVENTORY

Client_____
Date_____

ITEM	DESCRIPTION	RATING	DECIDE	ACTION
PANT	Blue jean with red patches	4	Fix	fixed

Rating: 1 = I hate it, 2 = Not crazy about it, 3 = Like it, 4 = Love it & keeping it
Decide: Keep, Fix, Clean, Toss, Donate

Step 2

WARDROBE PLANNER WORKSHEET

CLIENT NAME:

Step 1 Write an inventory of all clothing items client is keeping AFTER closet edit (any damaged, unwanted or inappropriate clothing tossed)

Blouses	Jackets	Tops	Pants	Jeans	Skirts	Dresses	Long Jackets

Step 3

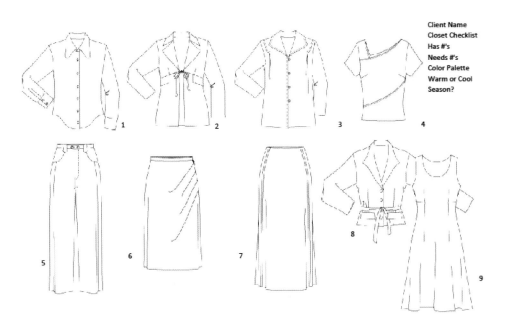

Client Name
Closet Checklist
Has #'s
Needs #'s
Color Palette
Warm or Cool
Season?

1) Blouse 2) Tie front jacket 3) Button front jacket does double duty as a blouse 4) Wrap top 5) Jean or plain pant
6) Skirt with detailing 7) Mid length skirt 8) Tie waist jacket 9) Sleeveless dress.
These 9 fashion basic pieces can be combined to create 42 separate outfits. Shown here are blanks. Just color in and go. For example - if your client
has these shapes in varying colors, prints and textures use copies of this sheet to help her organize outfits to wear.

This worksheet details the nine silhouettes you will need to create up to 42 separate outfits. Choose two or three colors from your existing wardrobe or purchase nine items in coordinating colors. You will have many outfits as a result.

Step 4

PLAN AN OUTFIT

Client Name: Description:	OUTFIT 1 Business Casual	OUTFIT 2 Business Dressy	OUTFIT 3 Business to Event	OUTFIT 4 Event
1 Blouse				
2 Jacket				
3 Jacket				
4 Top				
5 Pant				
6 Jean				
7 Skirt				
8 Skirt				
9 Dress				

ACCESSORY WORKSHEET

Client_____
Date_____

ACCESSORY/JEWEL	WEAR WITH	WHEN
gold necklace	white shirt. Grey pants	office
Pink scarf	Cream silk blouse/ black pants	Early Cocktail party

YOUR STYLE PERSONALITY

If you are like me you love to find out new things about yourself. I am always completing those 20 question lists you see in every other magazine around. I sometimes do the ones online just for fun.

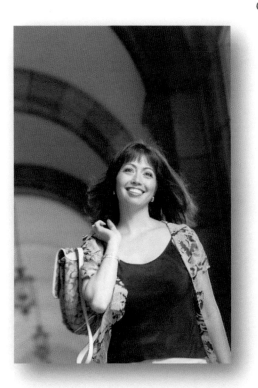

But I have yet to find a style personality questionnaire that defines my true tastes and synthesizes my likes and dislikes into one distinct style impression. So I developed my own and offer it to you to enjoy.

Think through the following questions before you answer them. Choose the answer that BEST describes how you dress NOW and what your style is like at this moment.

Defining your style personality will help you be more confident in your choices going forward. You will be able to identify the styles, lines and silhouettes of clothing that truly appeal to your personality. By sticking to your style personality a theme will emerge in your wardrobe and items will coordinate much easier when pulled together.

Your Style Personality can sometimes
be a mix of several, i.e.: **CONSERVATIVE** personalities
will sometimes want to mix things up and
add **CREATIVE** or **DRAMATIC** pieces to their look.

STYLE PERSONALITY DEFINED QUIZ

Circle each letter that seems the truest statement of your current style. Choose only ONE answer.

1)   I define my clothing choices as:

   a) Comfort first always
   b) I can't stand clutter. Everything must have a purpose
   c) My clothes have to be pretty – for casual, work or dressy occasions
   d) Aside from a few, around-the-house items, all my clothes make a statement
   e) The wackier, more diverse, more impossible the better
   f) Order and simplicity. Everything must be up-to-date and mix and match

2) I prefer work clothes that are:

   a) Separates that mix and match, comfortable yet smart
   b) Classically tailored clothes
   c) Preferably softer, fluid designs
   d) Bold combinations
   e) Individual but appropriate
   f) Elegantly blended neutral colors

3) For weekends I prefer

   a) Casual, relaxed gear
   b) A timeless, good quality skirt and sweater
   c) Pretty blouses and tops; nice shoes
   d) Something WOW
   e) Ethnic, avant-garde, unpredictable styling
   f) Simple but so chic

4) My best hairstyle is:

   a) Casual and windblown, natural
   b) Controlled and neat but not severe
   c) A soft, layered look, never short
   d) Something modern; my style changes all the time
   e) Spiky, loose curls; I use scarves and clips a lot
   f) Current, but timeless, in great condition

5) Fabrics I love include:

   a) Denim, knits, anything textured
   b) Natural fabrics; 100% wool, cotton, silk, organic
   c) Jersey, soft, lace, silk and vintage
   d) Rich velvets, brocades, suede's and corduroy
   e) Metallic's, leather, contrasting textures like tweed
   f) Best quality wool crepe, cashmere, linen, dupionis

6) The accessories I prefer:

   a) Not much, preferably natural beads and stones
   b) Pearls and gold
   c) Delicate chains and antique jewels
   d) Striking, bold pieces, one of a kind
   e) Ethnic; I like to layer them on
   f) Real jewels and quality costume, designer pieces

7) For evening I like to wear:

   a) A nice pantsuit
   b) Simple black dress, knee length
   c) A gorgeous dress with lots of detailing, vintage
   d) Colorful silk kimono or tunic with a skirt or pants
   e) Full length kimono with all the accessories
   f) Smoking jacket and matching trousers

8) My shoes are usually:

    a) Sneakers, high tops or walking shoes
    b) Flats or very low heels
    c) Higher heels with embellishments
    d) Smart boots or what's currently in style
    e) Funky styles, ballet flats to platforms
    f) A slight heel in a classic shape

9) My favorite colors are:

    a) Naturals, nothing bright or neon
    b) Blended colors but no bold colors
    c) Feminine pastels
    d) Rich and bold colors with black and white
    e) Neon, hand painted, brights
    f) Neutral colors, charcoal, pewter, ivory and cream

10) My style icons are:

    a) Katherine Hepburn, Marcia Cross, Diane Keaton
    b) Angelina Jolie, Victoria Beckham, Ivanka Trump
    c) Heidi Klum, Katie Holmes, Mary Kate Olson
    d) Cher, Rihanna, Janice Dickinson
    e) Tilda Swinton, Bjork, Madonna
    f) Michelle Obama, Brooke Shields, Nicole Kidman

11) When I shop:

    a) I spend as little time as possible
    b) I only buy when I need something new
    c) I buy clothes that I think others will like
    d) I buy the latest and greatest
    e) I am always looking for something no one else has
    f) I buy the best quality I can afford

Place a check mark in each box for each answer:

Question	A	B	C	D	E	F
1						
2						
3						
4						
5						
6						
7						
8						
9						
10						
11						
TOTAL						

- Enter and add the total amount of your answers in each column into the bottom row marked TOTAL.
- The column with the highest number of answers reveals your STYLE PERSONALITY – see below.

A. Conservative, Smart, Practical
B. Classic, Modern, Poise
C. Romantic, Vintage, Charming
D. Dramatic, Independent, Sexy
E. Artistic, Creative, Passionate
F. Elegant, Cultured, Classy

STYLE PERSONALITIES

Conservative, Smart, Practical

You love high quality fabrics such as tweeds, cashmeres and crisp pure cotton. Your look is Ivy League with a personal touch. You love wearing crisp white blouses paired with gray wool slacks and will add antique rhinestone and pearl jewels as a style stamp. You don't spend frivolously and your wardrobe is filled with conservative styles that will last the test of time. Your taste and choice in clothing mirrors most European women's.

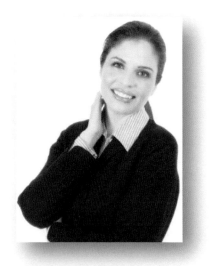

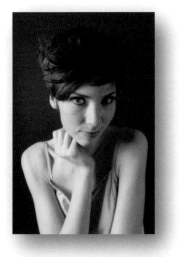

Classic, Modern, Poised

You also love quality fabrics but your clothing choices lean toward classic and elegant. Your color choices are always modern, for instance, you will buy a cashmere jacket in a gorgeous pink color. You look and feel great in Garbo pants with a tailored navy sailor jacket.

Romantic, Vintage, Charming

Soft ruffles, lace, antique buttons these are details you pay close attention to when choosing your clothing. You love to shop vintage clothing stores and have a stash of vintage slips you love to wear. Modern styles have to have romantic elements. You love hand-made and your jewelry matches this mood.

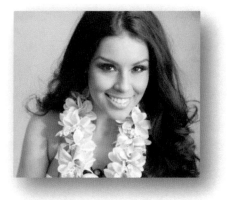

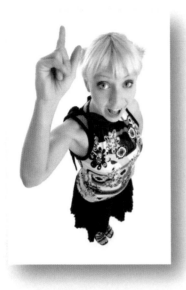

Dramatic, Independent, Sexy

Your clothing choices are always bold, confident and body conscious. You are not afraid to mix colors, patterns and styles from today's designers. You are in love with black lace and corsetry.

Artistic, Creative, Passionate

You, more than any other clothing personality, have an intense interest in color, texture, pattern and print and have the confidence to combine these elements in your dress and accessories. You always have the best shoes and bags.

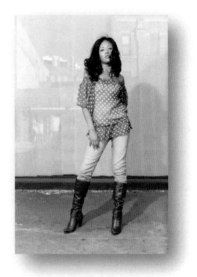

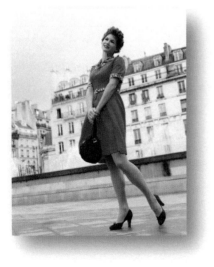

Elegant, Cultured, Classy

You are a couture fan and enjoy hand tailored clothing. Pearls and heirloom gold add dash to your cashmere jackets and silk trousers. You love wearing simple and elegant styles. IF you could you would wear 1930's fashion all the time.

EASY STEPS TO STYLE MASTERY

1. **Look behind you**: It is very important to review how you look before leaving your house. You never know, you might have tucked your jacket into your waistband, maybe you've spilled coffee down your tie or there is a big bleach spot on the back of those jeans. And, as happens more commonly, your clothing fit from behind looks awful. Always double check by holding a hand mirror and looking to see how good (or bad) your rear appears!

2. **Color-coordinate your outfits**: One of the easiest ways to color coordinate your clothing is to choose clothes in the same color family. For instance, wear a cream blouse with a cream skirt or a white blouse with cream pants. Likewise a gray jacket with black pants. Learn to work with neutrals. If you know how to use neutral colors as the base of your wardrobe, you can add color via accessories, bags, scarves, jewelry etc. Experts rely on color wheels to coordinate. If you do not own a color wheel go out and buy one. They save you time and money when learning to coordinate a chic wardrobe. To use effectively, choose neighboring colors on the wheel to coordinate outfits.

3. **Find a signature piece**: Pearls, scarves, hats, colors etc. these details can become your "signature". Many celebrities and style icons are memorable for their signatures and creating your own doesn't have to be difficult. You can start with something as simple as a colorful necklace. Does this signature (symbol) define your colorful personality perhaps? Do you see your "self" as romantic? Conservative? Casual? Sexy? Or dramatic? For example, Sophia Loren's style is dramatic. Her features are very prominent, her face distinctly Roman; her hourglass figure voluptuous and her personality passionate. Her signature "dramatic" look is a true reflection of who she is. Once you define your personality it's easy to find a signature to stamp your style.

4. **Tailor your clothes**: To create a chic look wear clothes that fit you perfectly. This requires you pay attention to detail. Sleeves need to be long enough, pants not too short, jackets fitted at the shoulder and waist, blouses tailored to your body shape. But be warned - when you buy off-the-rack clothing you run the risk of improper fit. I'm not saying don't buy off-the-rack, just that you will need a good tailor to fit them to your shape. Make sure the clothes you are wearing are comfortable otherwise you project discomfort and restlessness.

5. **Get a stylish hairstyle**: A little bit of research and a consultation with a great hairstylist will lead to the perfect haircut for your facial shape. Unless you're a quick study, you do not know your facial shape and without knowing it you'll never know which styles are flattering for you. Consulting with a pro is free. There are also on-line sites that help you determine your facial shape. You can try on virtual hairstyles suitable to your facial shape. As in clothing, your hairstyle should reflect your personality.

6. **Pay attention to details**: Your hair, your smile, how you feel when you wear a beautiful dress are little, but important, details that help you feel confident, empowered and positive. Paying attention to details is not just about whether your buttons are buttoned, your snaps are snapped, or your belt is belted; it's about the relevancy of detail: from beautiful buttons, quality belts and fabrications, to excellent tailoring and fit. And, don't forget accessory details - socks should match your shoes and pants, your handbag style should be congruent with your clothes etc.

7. **Wear good jewels**: I recently reviewed an international publication's best-dressed list. What caught my eye was that each of these best-dressed women wore important jewelry. Chic jewelry does not have to be a big investment but an investment in chic-ness is always great. Three strands of pearls, a gold cable chain necklace, an elegant watch or a pair

of pearl (or gold) earrings are all you actually need to look chic. Costume jewelry is rarely chic (unless it's vintage). Stick with the classics, and you cannot go wrong.

8. **Speak Chic**: Many chic women I know are multilingual. When they converse in English they throw in a few native words for effect. If English is your only language it's still easy to incorporate foreign words into your conversation. This will make you seem incredibly chic, worldly and accomplished. Compare how *"I love the way you look"* sounds to *"J'adore how you look"* and you'll hear what I mean! Be natural, have fun with it so it does not seem contrived, just playful and cosmopolitan.

9. **Manners and etiquette**: These are at the heart of what chic is. If your manners and etiquette skills are impeccable you can get by with a relaxed appearance. However, for our purposes (creating a chic look) let's agree that manners, perfect etiquette and a chic appearance add up to one very chic woman. These days there are so many etiquette professionals and classes, both in person and online, that no one can use the excuse that they never learned how to be socially appropriate. To me perfect manners transcend other imperfections. If your manners are perfect you are too!

10. **Be Charming**: Charm is one of the most important aspects of a woman's personality and one of the greatest contributors to being chic. When you can turn on the charm and incorporate it into your overall image then you will be chic. Even in this world of "all business, all the time" don't fear using your feminine charms. Best dressed women always rely on charm as the path to chic-ness!

HAIRSTYLES AND FACE SHAPES

Your hairstyle is an important part of your overall image. By getting your hair cut and styled to suit your face, you will get the look that is the most flattering for you. You might be surprised at how very different you can look with the right hairstyle. Finding the right hairstyle to suit your face is often challenging. You have to balance the current trends with what will look best on you. But how do you know what will make you look your best?

Figure Out Your Face Shape

In order to find the right hairstyle for your face, you first want to determine your face shape. Here is a brief guide (also reference "Face Shapes" on page 70 for more information):

- *Oval*: This type of face is egg-shaped and equal in size on top and bottom. An oval is the ideal facial shape because it can support many flattering types of jewelry and hairstyles.
- *Heart*: Wider at the temples and narrower at the chin.
- *Round*: This face type is similar to the oval, but shorter and wider.
- *Triangle*: The opposite of the heart, this type of face is usually wide at the chin with a narrow forehead. Characterizes by a prominent, wide jaw line.
- *Square*: A strong jaw and squared-off features are typical of this type.
- *Rectangle*: A longer version of the square face.

Go Long to Slim the Face

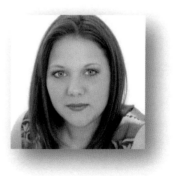

For round faces, the worst thing you can do is to get a chin length cut. That will just draw attention to the roundness of the face. To make your face look longer and slimmer, keep hair long, at least shoulder length. While some layering at the bottom can work, it is usually best to keep layers out of the face and below the jaw line. Longer styles also go very well with an oval-shaped face.

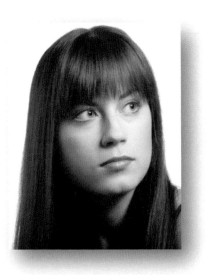

Use Bangs to Hide Flaws

Bangs camouflage a large forehead or are often used to soften a face. Bangs usually look best when they are not too full, so stick to just a light coverage. Bangs go well with heart-shaped faces to minimize the width of the forehead, and are also ideal for softening a square or rectangular face. Avoid using them with a round face shape, since this will cut off length and make the face look even shorter.

Layers Create Softness

When you have straight lines in your face, such as those with a square or rectangular face, some well-placed layers can really help soften your face and create a more feminine look. Be careful of having too many layers, since this can actually start to look frizzy and unkempt, but a handful of wisps looks great.

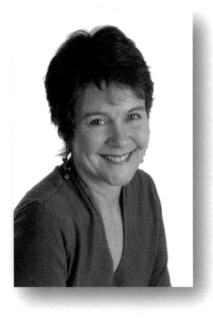

Short Hairstyles Add Width to the Jaw

Obviously, if you already have a naturally wide chin, you won't want to opt for a bob or any other chin-length cut. However, for heart-shaped faces, this is the ideal hairstyle to balance out the wide forehead. Short hair can also be used successfully with a rectangular face, to create a shorter look, particularly if combined with a layered cut to add texture and softness to the face.

Add Some Curl For Extra Body

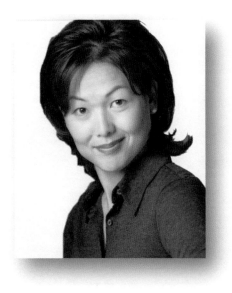

Not everyone is blessed with full hair and when you have a triangular or a rectangular face, a little extra volume can really help. Going with a light perm or curl can help add some volume to your hair and balance out these face types.

Now that you have a fairly good idea of what your face shape is and which hairstyles compliment it, you can take a look at a variety of hairstyles from magazines, the Internet or hairstylists' style books and decide which is the right one for your face. Choosing the best hairstyle for you will result in a great look that enhances your natural beauty and makes you feel your best everyday.

A hairstyle is the frame for the face.
A great haircut will showcase
your MOST important facial feature
– your eyes.

ACCESSORY SUCCESS

To find your signature accessory first know your style personality (see Style Personality Defined Questionaire). If you are conservative then stick to conservative patterns, classic styling and high quality items. Pearl necklaces or silk Hermès scarves fit the bill for you.

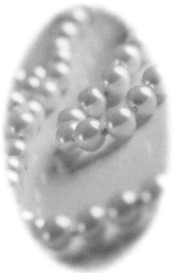

If you are a romantic then you would choose floral or delicate prints and fabrics for scarves, shawls or jackets. Your jewels would be old-fashioned in nature; cameos on velvet ribbons or perhaps delicate pearls twined round your neck several times.

The important aspect of picking a signature accessory is that it must be congruent with your style personality and as such will match your clothing styles.

Hairstyles, accessories and jewels are important components of your individual style, but it is the details that make the difference between unfashionable and fashionable women. For instance, fashionable women pay strict attention to even the tiniest of details, up to and including the color of the laces of their boots but will not go as far as to match their bags with their shoes.

Fashionable women look at the whole picture of the outfit they wear and see a portrait of style rather than individual pieces of a whole. Try to keep this in mind the next time you pull your outfit together, look at the whole picture as a portrait of style from the color of your shoe laces to the earrings on your earlobes.

Define The Look Of The Outfit

As you choose what top to wear with your pants start to think of a "portrait" or a "concept" in your style. Are you polished? Perhaps going for a 1940's look? How about an oriental feel to today's look? Begin with an idea in mind and then:

Build on it: Keep adding layers - a jacket, maybe an additional piece such as a vest or shawl. Stay consistent with the color palette or print family you are working in.

Edit: As you view yourself in the mirror keep a critical eye to the story you are creating and pull back or add on. Erase or embellish.

Refine: Now pull back some more or add one more piece and again, step back from the mirror, turn and view yourself from all angles (backside included).

Accent: Once you have scanned yourself front, side and back then you are ready to add the final touches - the accent of accessories. This is when you would, as a painter does, put the final finishing touches to your portrait - earrings to match your eye shade or perhaps a pair of shoes to blend with the color of your skirt. As Stacy London says "think about what goes, not about what matches".

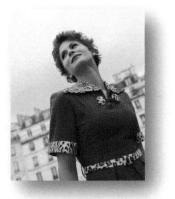

Review: View yourself one last time in the mirror and ask yourself if the portrait is now finished. If so then ask yourself what the mood is? Romantic, smart, sexy, audacious, calm etc.? Once you have determined the mood THEN choose a perfume to match but only apply a tiny amount. Just a drop is all you need to complete your work of art.

JEWELS TO MATCH FACIAL SHAPES

Pearls, gold, diamonds? Fine jewelry, costume jewelry, handmade or antique? With so many choices available it might seem daunting to decide which jewels work for your style personality.

Chic jewelry will define your taste so keep it simple. A fantastic pearl necklace, classic gold link choker or simple diamond drop pendant necklace suffice for a jewelry wardrobe. A quality pair of pearl earrings, a pair of diamond studs or a pair of simple gold hoops are also a good addition to your collection.

When you stick to the classics of pearl, gold, diamond or gemstone you can build your wardrobe around them. Also, you don't have to spend a fortune for a good piece of jewelry, just pay attention to how it's made, what it's made of and if you like the styling.

If you don't already know your face shape read the following guide, then you will be able to choose jewels that flatter your particular shape.

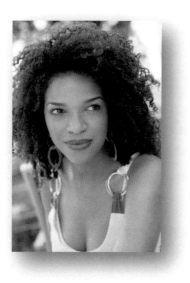

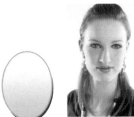

OVAL FACIAL SHAPE - This facial shape is egg shaped. It can also be a long oval, think of a long oval as an elongated egg shape. This face shape is equal in size across the face horizontally and down the face vertically and as such is perfectly proportioned. If you have this type of facial shape you can wear many styles, shapes and sizes of earrings, necklaces, scarves and hats.

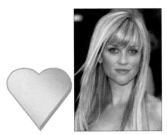

HEART SHAPE is wider at the temples and tapers to a smaller almost pointy chin. Across the face from ear to ear is one width and from hairline to chin length is longer. Faces in this shape can be proportionally balanced by wearing jewelry styles that elogate the face. Earrings can be long drops in angular shapes for maximum flatter!

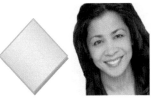

DIAMOND FACIAL SHAPE - Women with this facial shape have wide jawlines that stretch out to their ears. Typically they have wonderful cheekbones. To proportion this facial shape with jewelry seek to balance out the width by increasing visual length. Long drop shaped earrings will flatter a diamond shape, as will long necklaces and scarves tied below the collar bone.

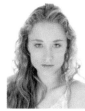

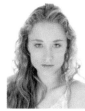SQUARE FACIAL SHAPE - Face shape is angular and equally as wide at the forehead, jawline and cheekbones. To proportion the face with jewelry choose earring styles that draw attention vertically across cheeks continuing down the neck.   Large chandelier shaped earrings work well for this purpose.

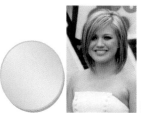

ROUND FACIAL SHAPE - This particular shape is wide throughout the jaw and cheek area, almost a filled out oval shape and can wear many styles of earring and necklace as long as the proportion of visual interest is vertical (to elongate the face) and not horizontal (which will widen the face).

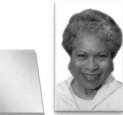

TRIANGLE FACIAL SHAPE has a wider jawline and narrower temple. The best jewels are ones that when worn will widen the face at the cheekbone. Earrings that are dramatic, bold and big and worn close to the ear are the most flattering for this facial shape. The best neckwear can include long necklaces to elongate the neck. Chokers and wrapped scarves do not flatter this facial shape.

Sketch your facial shape here and compare with the above shapes:

SPEECH and COMMUNICATION

I once met a woman in Europe who looked incredibly well groomed. She dressed in wonderful avant garde designer outfits that flattered her body shape. Her hair was always coiffed and her poise beyond reproach BUT she had the loudest voice this side of New York! Her voice threw her carefully prepared image out the door and, while first impressions are all important, it is the second impression that, if negative, leaves a lasting impression too.

Speech refers to the act of delivering a spoken communication. Whether one delivers softly, succinctly or brashly and crudely the listener can be affected positively or negatively. Therefore your choice of speech can greatly affect your business dealings and social interactions. Choose your speech carefully and learn to refine any anomalies in the way you speak.

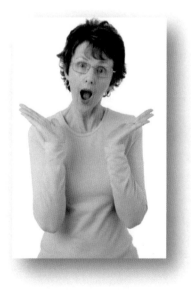

Learn to speak-chic. By this I mean choose your words carefully and deliver them slowly, elegantly and with ease. When people whose first language is not English speak they tend to choose their words carefully and enunciate them slowly. This creates a sense of refinement in their manner and is quite pleasant to observe. Even if English is your first language you can still practice speaking slowly, clearly and with charm.

When you communicate you want to convey confidence and credibility, and you want people to feel compelled to listen. Considering that a lot of what is communicated is non-verbal, body language and vocal inflection can miss-communicate your real message. Use these seven tips to increase the effectiveness of your communication and ensure that you always get your point across.

Recognize the Power in Your Posture

Your communication starts with the stance you choose when you speak. Whether you are talking on the phone or you are in a meeting, it is always best to stand up when you speak. To really get your point across pull your shoulders back to slightly exaggerate your posture and open up your diaphragm. Do not play with a pen, fidget or cross your arms and legs when you speak. Using open body language conveys that you mean what you say and are open to the input of others.

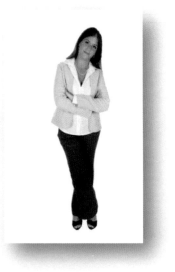

Project Your Voice

Recognize that the purpose of the volume of your voice is not exclusively to ensure that the listeners hear you. Volume adds authority to your vocal presentation and it is important to speak up to project volume if that is what the situation demands. Remember to use volume only when appropriate – don't be an inconsiderate 'loud mouth'.

Be Articulate

The most prevalent challenge in every day communication is the lack of clear articulation in conversation. Every time you use a speech filler as in "ah" or "um" or "you know" or "so," you are detracting from the confidence you want your words to convey and you diminish the power of your message. Ask a trusted colleague or friend to tell you what your speech fillers are and work to eliminate them. You can also record yourself on the phone; you will be surprised at what you hear.

Remember to be clear about the message you are delivering. Don't cloud the issues you are talking about. If you are delivering a message about appropriate office attire, you don't want to start giving detailed messages about the upcoming company picnic.

Pay Attention to Your Pace

Everyone has their own natural pace for speaking. When we are nervous many people really speed up. When we talk too fast we convey a lack of experience, and we do not allow time for our listeners to comprehend what we are saying. Pay attention to your pace, be sure to breathe and do not be afraid to pause.

Keep In Eye Contact

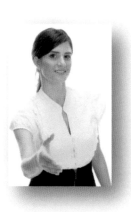

Another huge challenge many people have when they are talking is that they look everywhere except at the people to whom they are speaking. Do not let that be you. When you avoid looking at people, they may subconsciously feel that you are not telling the truth and you are also more likely to lose their attention. Staying in eye contact makes people feel like you are speaking to them personally rather than just speaking out loud.

Be Prepared Even When You Think It's Not Necessary

So often women think that because they know their work or their projects so well that they can "wing" a briefing or even a fairly long report or presentation. Don't do it. Winging it never works well unless you have delivered the same message or report or presentation a hundred times. Take five minutes to figure out your talking points, or take even longer for a major presentation. Preparation makes you feel confident and ensures your nerves will not get the best of you. Even before you call a client or leave a message for your boss do not hesitate to take a few moments to jot down your ideas. This way you will always come across as the competent professional that you are.

Be Consistent

Keep your message consistent. Don't contradict yourself from one communication to the next, or be inconsistent in your words on the same subject to different people. This can quickly put your coworkers in the position of distrusting you. Consistent communication is key to building confidence in the workplace.

Every time you speak you solidify or confuse the effective image you have been working hard to create. Identify which of these communication areas need the most attention from you and get started today. Your communication is the cornerstone of your image. Make sure yours is working for you.

YOUR NON-VERBAL COMMUNICATION STYLE

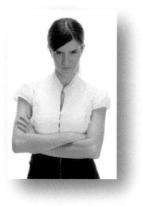

The following non-verbal communication points provide you an opportunity to self-edit. Rate yourself and make comments about your observations based on the subtle (and not so subtle) messages you are sending regarding your image and appearance. If you can't be objective have a friend or a trusted associate review these points with you.

BODY LANGUAGE

Stance (i.e.: confident, shy etc):

Posture (excellent, needs work, poor etc):

Greeting style (reserved, emotional, friendly etc):

Eye contact (shape of eyes, low/medium/high contact):

Handshake (loose, too soft, firm, too firm):

Voice (tone, quality, and pitch):

Language (accent, inflection, ability for small talk):

Eye movement when in conversation:

Body language (reflexive/non-reflexive/natural or forced)?

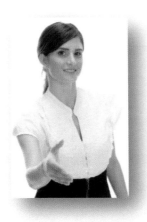

IMAGE REVIEW

Rate yourself on these points which ask how you are seen by others; note how your visual appearance conveys instant messages about you to viewers.

Poise:

Manners:

Fashion style (defined, distinct, individual, confident etc):

Communication component of dress (frazzled, clean, messy etc):

Messages of appearance (economic, social, cultural):

Energy level (mellow, depressed, hyper etc):

Choice of color in clothing:

Mannerisms or ticks:

Body odor:

Emotional expressions:

Facial expressions:

IMAGE REVIEW—CONTINUED

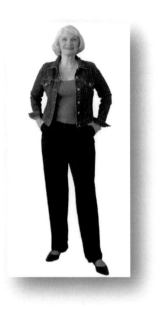

Quality of accessories:

Labels or brands represented:

Grooming:

Makeup:

Body modifications (tattoos, piercings etc):

Smile quality:

Self-esteem:

Body confidence:

Other observations:

Did you notice areas that need adjustment or change? If so, then set about making the appropriate changes to your image immediately. After all the messages you are sending have an impact on how others treat you.

If you could change ONE thing
about your image, right now,
what would it be? Don't think too
hard about this task; just do
the first thing that comes to mind.

ETIQUETTE and CHARM

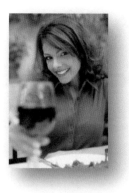

Since we can't cover the entire world of manners and etiquette in this book, suffice to say that if you do need help in this area there are many resources at your disposal. There are protocol schools and etiquette classes you can attend. There are also many how-to articles available on the World Wide Web. Regardless of where you live, the universal principals of good manners, civility and appropriate etiquette always apply in your interactions with others.

The point is that when you school yourself in appropriate customs, protocol, manners and etiquette you reveal yourself to be a woman of style and substance. Your interactions with others will be rife with ease and confidence and you will make a wonderful impression wherever you are. Take the time to polish your skills in manners and etiquette and your influence in social and business situations will thrive.

I once read that "charm is the way of getting the answer 'yes' without asking a clear question" (Albert Camus). Charm is one of a woman's greatest strengths. The power of charm is irrefutable and easily put into practice by most of us. Without charm a woman just isn't fully present. With charm she is all she can be. That doesn't mean to say that charm should be used for manipulation, something entirely different from charm. Audrey Hepburn comes to mind when I think of charm. She had a distinct personality steeped in adorable quirks of being. This is an important distinction about charm - it is different for each woman because it depends so much of individual personality.

To be able to delight others with pleasant conversation, a joyful disposition, a sunny outlook on life, these are all aspects of charm. Learn to cultivate this quality in yourself, to use it as a symbol of chic-ness in your world. Remember that charm is a large part of external appearances and attraction. Use charm to paint your personal style portrait then watch the world take notice.

ETIQUETTE SUCCESS

What is poise? What is the difference between business etiquette and social etiquette? What is charm and how does it have the power to influence people? As one of the most important communication skills one can master, etiquette ranks at the top. Social faux pas are rampant in today's world both in the business environment and the social milieu. It is imperative to learn how to be confident and socially comfortable in all situations whether social or business related. Being skilled in etiquette and manners takes you a long way toward personal comfort while interacting with others.

There are many aspects to a person's non-verbal communication and etiquette skills that can be improved upon. The following are just a few aspects of etiquette for you to review. If you feel deficient in any one area you might consider taking a class. Many local community colleges offer programs and courses. Check out what's available in your neighborhood with a quick online search.

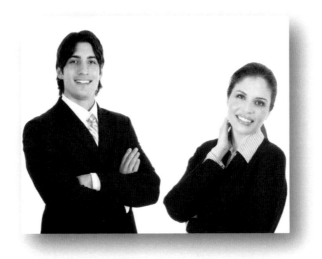

- Poise and Presence
- Perfect Posture
- Social Confidence
- Social Civility
- Language Usage
- Mannerism Awareness
- Charm & Sophistication
- Visual Poise for Social Affairs
- Handling Parties
- The "Thank You" Letter
- Your Self Confidence

Poise also relates to posture. How you hold your body says a lot about how much you care about yourself. An erect spine will help you breathe better, so, when you are about to make that important speech, stand tall!

MAKEUP

Makeup affords women a simple, effective and inexpensive way to dramatically enhance or change our appearance.

The right makeup color and application can make us positively glow, while the wrong makeup color or application can ruin an otherwise perfect look.

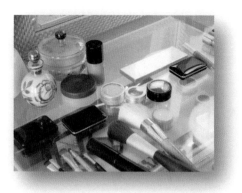

This guide will take you through the basic steps of makeup application, and then give you some guidelines for selecting your makeup colors and tools. At the back of this chapter you will find a face chart to use when testing makeup at the makeup counter.

A woman doesn't always have to look glamorous when going out, but a few touches of make-up here and there are more than enough to make your face stand out.

YOUR FACE IN TEN STEPS

Makeup application done well can take years off your face and make you look and feel wonderful. This guide is simplified into 10 steps. Making up your face should take you about 5 to 10 minutes at the most. Simple, perfectly applied makeup can help you put together a polished working image. A stylish, balanced look will make you feel really confident and ready to face the day.

STEP ONE/ CONCEALER

Concealer's are a fast and effective way to cover up lines, spots or shadows. Use them to hide scars, blotches or veins, not just to get perfect looking skin but to build a canvas on which to paint in the rest of your makeup.

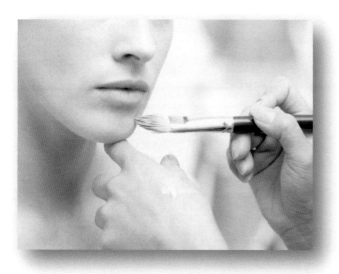

Corrective concealer's are a concentrated form of foundation and come is a range for colors. Find one that matches your skin tone.

Color concealer's typically come in 3 color choices- green, yellow, and **lavender** (mauve). You need to understand which color concealer will neutralize the flaw. Look at the flaw you want to cover. What color is it? Is it acne (red) or under-eye circles (blue)? By identifying this first, you are now ready to conceal those nasty little imperfections! Here's a list of color concealer's and what they neutralize:

Yellow concealer:

Use to conceal bluish bruises, under-eye circles and mild red tones on the face.

Lavender concealer:

Use to normalize yellow-colored skin imperfections such as sallow complexions and yellow bruises. It can also help conceal very dark under-eye circles and dark spots on bronze skin tones.

Green concealer:

Use to neutralize red tones on the skin. Use green concealer for covering blemishes, pimples, red blotches, rosacea, port-wine stains.

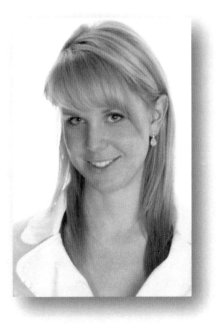

STEP TWO/ FOUNDATION

Foundation is well named - it is the base upon which your face is painted. Once your foundation is applied your skin as canvas is ready to paint!

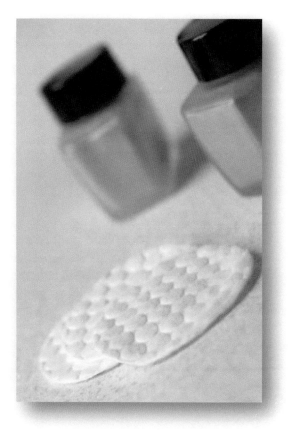

Foundation comes in a cream, liquid, or cake form. If you have oily skin use water based liquid and apply with a sponge. If your skin is normal with dry spots use an oil based foundation. Be careful to match your foundation (also known as base) to the skin along your jaw line. Apply a small dot of foundation, blend in to the skin and if you can't see the makeup after you have blended it in, then that's the right shade for you. Do this test under lighting and in front of a mirror.

Do's and Don'ts for applying foundation:

- Don't apply foundation to dirty or sweaty skin as this will clog pores and encourage pimples and acne.
- Don't apply foundation to your neck area as the skin here is thinner and not the same shade as your face. You will be two toned and, besides that, you run the risk of getting makeup on your clothing.
- Do apply just enough so that your concealer is concealed. Too much foundation and all your wrinkles will start to show.
- Don't apply foundation to skin that is breaking out. If you have to wear foundation choose a medicated or custom blended product that contains natural and mineral ingredients.

- Do apply foundation in *up and out* strokes using a sponge applicator. Rinse these applicators between foundation applications but do not use soap as this will irritate your skin the next time you apply your base.

> Test foundation on the inside of the forearm where the skin tone color is closest to the color on the neck near your face. Makeup should blend with the skin of the neck and jawbone.

STEP THREE/ POWDER

Powder gives your face an even-ness and, if applied properly, a healthy sheen. It also sets your foundation so it stays put and looks good longer. It is a final layer to concealing lines or skin blemishes that concealer and foundation aren't able to cover.

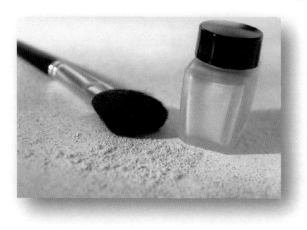

A translucent or colorless powder is the best. A mineral based powder even better. Powders come in pressed or loose form. You will need to use a powder brush to apply either form. Loose powder gives the best coverage and lasts longer. Dust it lightly over your entire face then shake off any excess powder and brush over your face one more time to blend.

Pressed powders come in compact form, sometimes with individual applicators. DO NOT use these applicators. They are usually cotton or synthetic fabric and will remove your concealer and base foundation. Always use a powder brush (large and soft) to apply powders.

Choose a skin tone match the same way you do with foundation - by applying a small amount of powder to your jaw line and watching how it disappears with your skin tone.

Apply powder in downward strokes and follow the way your facial hair grows to avoid lumps and clumps.

STEP FOUR/ BLUSH

Blush is applied to create a youthful, healthy look. Indeed, it is applied to the apples of the cheeks to give a fresh scrubbed "natural" glow to the skin. Blush comes in powder or cake form and is always applied with a brush, never a sponge. Use blush sparingly as a little goes a long way.

Powder blush - this should be applied over your foundation. Dip your brush, tap off excess, and make a smile. Where the apples of your cheek lift is where you apply the blush. Move in an upward motion toward your outer eye. Blend a few times making sure that the color looks natural.

Cream blusher - applying cream blusher breaks the rules of makeup and is one of only a few times when you will use your fingers to apply color. Start with a small dab of blush and apply to the apple of your cheek. Blend, blend, and blend to get a soft glow. Again, you do not want to see the blush sitting on your face. It must blend in. You can also use a foundation sponge wedge instead of fingers.

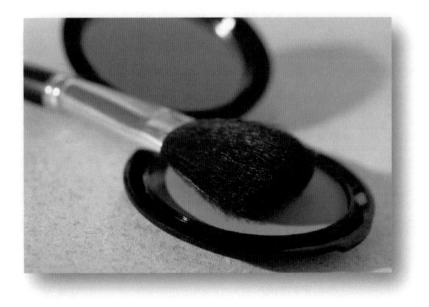

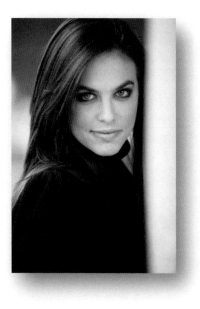

Color choices:

To gauge your best makeup colors you'll need to take a look at the underlying skin shade of your face. If you haven't already had your colors analyzed the easiest way to discover if you are cool based or warm based undertone is to test at the makeup counter. Makeup artists can diagnose you swiftly.

YOUR COLORING	YOUR MAKEUP FAMILY
Dark Hair / Olive Skin	Warm Brown
Red Hair / Warm Skin	Warm Peach
Red Hair / Cool Skin	Soft Peach
Dark Hair / Warm Skin	Rosy Brown
Dark Hair / Cool Skin	Cool Rose
Blonde Hair / Warm Skin	Tawny Pink
Blond Hair / Cool Skin	Baby Pink

STEP 5/ EYEBROWS

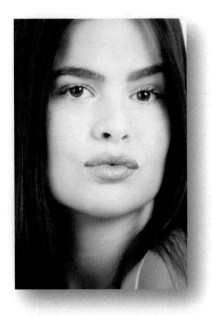

Eyebrows are the frames of the eyes and need your attention. Usually neglected, over plucked and sometimes shaved, the eyebrow has the power to make your face come alive with personality. Take a lesson is plucking, or get them professionally shaped.

To define your eyebrows use a pencil or powder applied with an eyebrow brush. Have your eyebrow comb ready to finish with gel. The gel will set the eyebrows in place. Ideally you should use a slanted (angled) brush for eyebrows.

Start by combing the eyebrow hairs down. Find the top of the eyebrow arch. Dip your angled brush into powder and starting at the arch draw a line of powder across the top of the eyebrow down toward the outer eye. Dip the brush a second time and make another line (or two) from the beginning of your eyebrow nearer to the nose and draw in to meet the arch line.

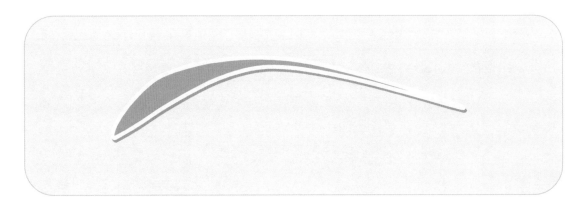

STEP 6/ EYESHADOW

Eye shadow comes in powder, stick, liquid and cream form. You can also have it applied via airbrush!

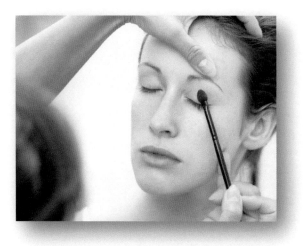

Powder eye shadows are the most popular and come in pressed powder containers usually with an applicator. Do not use the applicator. Instead use one of your brushes. Using a damp sponge head applicator for powders will make them darker - perfect for evening looks.

- Start with a neutral ivory powder on your sponge applicator.
- Sweep it over your lid and out toward the outer eye. This is your base eye makeup.
- Using another, smaller sponge head applicator, apply a medium dark color into the fold of your eye lid.
- Then take a larger brush and apply a highlight color to the brow bone under your eyebrow.
- Use a liquid liner for the lid and then sweep a final brush of neutral powder over your lid.

STEP 7/ EYELINER

Eyeliner also comes in liquid, powder or pencil form. You can even find it in felt-tip pen! You can use several types on your upper lids. For your lower lids (under your lower eyelashes) it's best to use cream pencil for easy smudging. You can apply eyeliner either with sharp edges or with soft and smoky edges.

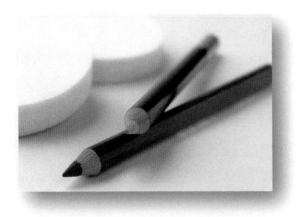

- Looking down into a mirror and keeping your hand steady, apply liquid eyeliner along your upper lashes.

- Use a clean cotton swab to work some brown eye shadow under your lower lashes to add some subtle definition.

- The perfect eyeliner is one that matches the color in the outer ring of the iris in your eye.

- Eyeliner defines the eyes and can make them look smaller. If your eyes are already on the small side just apply liner to the upper lashes and not the lower.

- Close set eyes do better when the lines are smudged and applied from the center of the lashes out toward the eye corner.

STEP 8/ MASCARA

Mascara is an invaluable way to create a flattering frame for the eyes. Most mascara come in a wand like applicator and are easy to apply to the lashes. There are many varieties of lash thickening mascara on the market these days many in colors like blue, green, gold and even red! This favorite tool of women can be found in most makeup bags.

Start by applying mascara to your upper lashes. Brush the tops down to the tips and then brush from the bottom of the lash to the tips. Repeat this step for your bottom lashes. To fill in any missing lashes take the wand and with zigzag motions move it over the top lashes and then the lower lashes.

Wait a few seconds for the mascara to dry and then blink. If any clumps appear use a Q-tip™ cotton swab and gently smooth out the lashes.

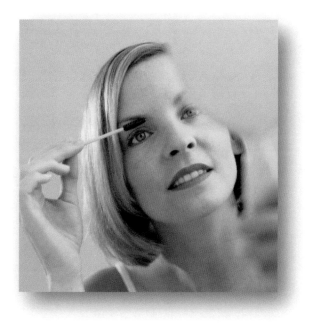

STEP 9/ LIP LINER

Lip liners are used to provide an outline for your lips prior to applying lipstick or lip gloss. Liner should be applied to treated lips. Use a clear matte lip salve to prepare your lip. Apply the liner to the entire outer line of your lip. Lip liner can also be used to camouflage or correct miss-shaped or irregular shaped lips.

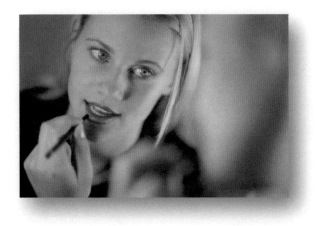

- Use the lip liner to draw the outer silhouette and your lipstick to fill in the color. It's important to match your lip liner as closely as possible with your lipstick.

- Applying lip liner to the entire lip area keeps lips colored even when your lipstick wears off.

- Outline your lips with a color slightly darker than your shade of lipstick.

- Use color to create the illusion of fuller lips by darkening the edges of the lips.

- To define downward sloping lips draw lip liner slightly higher on the upper lip.

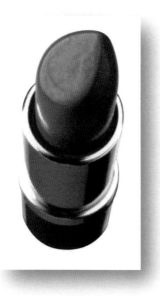

STEP 10/ LIPSTICK

Lipstick is the easiest and fastest way to give your face a splash of color. Lipsticks come in bullet form, pot of color, gloss and brush on. Lipsticks in bullet form are the most popular way to use lip color. The more pigment in a lipstick the longer it will last on your lips. Use your lip brush to apply and carefully paint on color.

Gloss can also be applied using a brush. You can use gloss alone or to top off your lipstick.

- Prime your lips with clear matte lip salve (balm).

- Apply lip liner first – apply around the edges of the lips first, then color in the entire lip area. This keeps your lips colored even after lipstick wears off.

- Stroke your lip brush over the tip of the lipstick, pick up color and get ready to paint your lips.

- Draw your lips tight over your teeth in a forced smile.

- Fill in the outline you created with the lip liner with the lipstick color for a shiny finish.

- Dab with a Kleenex™ or top with lip gloss.

FACE PLAY - LIST YOUR PERSONAL COLORS HERE:

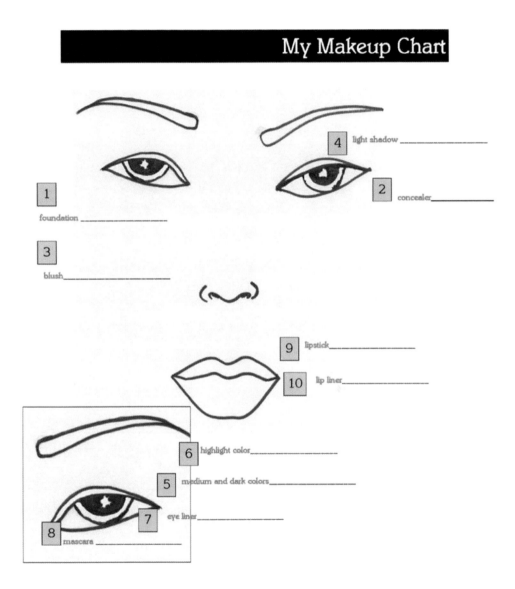

My Makeup Chart

4   light shadow _____

1   2   concealer_____

foundation _____

3

blush_____

9   lipstick_____

10   lip liner_____

6   highlight color_____

5   medium and dark colors_____

7   eye liner_____

8   mascara _____

BRUSH UP YOUR MAKEUP

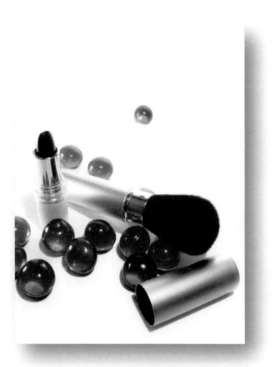

Successful make-up application depends on the tools you use. While it's fine to use your fingertips for some jobs it's always better to use proper tools. Here is a list of basic makeup tools you will need to get a professional finish.

Make-up sponge - *natural wedge shaped ones*

Powder brush - *large soft (preferably sable)*

Blusher brush - *slightly smaller than powder brush*

Eye shadow brush - *soft tip, rounded brush*

Eye shadow sponge - *sponge top applicator*

Eyelash brush/comb combo - *course hair with plastic comb*

Lip brush - *retractable with cover preferred*

Eyelash curlers - *choose a professional quality curler*

ATTITUDE

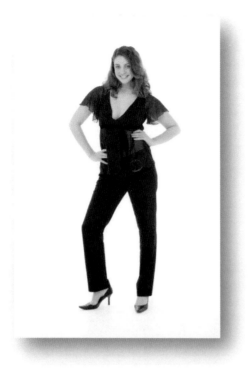

Let's finish this book with a word about attitude.

Definition: A position of the body or manner of carrying oneself: stood in a graceful attitude. A state of mind or a feeling; disposition: had a positive attitude about work.

When it comes to your image and dressing well, attitude goes a long way toward projecting confidence. Attitude is about your stance, your choices of dress and your personality. It can make or break a job interview, a client meeting, a sales pitch or a first date. Be sure your attitude is appropriate to the situation you are in and be equally sure that your appearance matches your attitude.

You're now well on your way to *"Mastering The Art Of Dressing Well"*. After reading this book you know the basics and then some. All you need to do now is create your own style and look, one that is appropriate for the world you live in. Be sure to stay true to who you are, always wear comfortable clothing and project confidence so you can make that all important, great, first impression. Now you are ready to take a new look at **your look** and use your appearance to your advantage.

HOURGLASS BODYSHAPE

BUST				WAIST				HIPS		
48	TO	50		36	TO	40		48	TO	50
47	TO	49		35	TO	39		47	TO	49
46	TO	48		34	TO	38		46	TO	48
45	TO	47		33	TO	37		45	TO	47
44	TO	46		32	TO	36		44	TO	46
43	TO	45		31	TO	35		43	TO	45
42	TO	44		30	TO	34		42	TO	44
41	TO	43		29	TO	33		41	TO	43
40	TO	42		28	TO	32		40	TO	42
39	TO	41		27	TO	31		39	TO	41
38	TO	40		26	TO	30		38	TO	40
37	TO	39		25	TO	29		37	TO	39
36	TO	38		24	TO	28		36	TO	38
35	TO	37		23	TO	27		35	TO	37
34	TO	36		22	TO	26		34	TO	36
33	TO	35		21	TO	25		33	TO	35
32	TO	34		20	TO	24		32	TO	34
31	TO	33		19	TO	23		31	TO	33
30	TO	32		18	TO	22		30	TO	32
29	TO	31		17	TO	21		29	TO	31
28	TO	30		16	TO	20		28	TO	30
27	TO	29		15	TO	19		27	TO	29
26	TO	28		14	TO	18		26	TO	28
25	TO	27		13	TO	17		25	TO	27
24	TO	26		12	TO	16		24	TO	26

Hold ruler in a straight line across this chart. If clients measurements do not align straight across then move to the next chart and so on until you determine actual body shape.

INVERTED TRIANGLE BODY SHAPE

BUST				WAIST				HIPS		
48	TO	51		43	TO	46		43	TO	46
47	TO	50		42	TO	45		42	TO	45
46	TO	49		41	TO	44		41	TO	44
45	TO	48		40	TO	43		40	TO	43
44	TO	47		39	TO	42		39	TO	42
43	TO	46		38	TO	41		38	TO	41
42	TO	45		37	TO	40		37	TO	40
41	TO	44		36	TO	39		36	TO	39
40	TO	43		35	TO	38		35	TO	38
39	TO	42		34	TO	37		34	TO	37
38	TO	41		33	TO	36		33	TO	36
37	TO	40		32	TO	35		32	TO	35
36	TO	39		31	TO	34		31	TO	34
35	TO	38		30	TO	33		30	TO	33
34	TO	37		29	TO	32		29	TO	32
33	TO	36		28	TO	31		28	TO	31
32	TO	35		27	TO	30		27	TO	30
31	TO	34		26	TO	29		26	TO	29
30	TO	33		25	TO	28		25	TO	28
29	TO	32		24	TO	27		24	TO	27
28	TO	31		23	TO	26		23	TO	26
27	TO	30		22	TO	25		22	TO	25
26	TO	29		21	TO	24		21	TO	24
25	TO	28		20	TO	23		20	TO	23
24	TO	27		19	TO	22		19	TO	22

Hold ruler in a straight line across this chart. If clients measurements do not align straight across then move to the next chart and so on until you determine actual body shape.

RECTANGLE BODYSHAPE

BUST				WAIST				HIPS		
48	TO	51		45	TO	48		47	TO	50
47	TO	50		44	TO	47		46	TO	49
46	TO	49		43	TO	46		45	TO	48
45	TO	48		42	TO	45		44	TO	47
44	TO	47		41	TO	44		43	TO	46
43	TO	46		40	TO	43		42	TO	45
42	TO	45		39	TO	42		41	TO	44
41	TO	44		38	TO	41		40	TO	43
40	TO	43		37	TO	40		39	TO	42
39	TO	42		36	TO	39		38	TO	41
38	TO	41		35	TO	38		37	TO	40
37	TO	40		34	TO	37		36	TO	39
36	TO	39		33	TO	36		35	TO	38
35	TO	38		32	TO	35		34	TO	37
34	TO	37		31	TO	34		33	TO	36
33	TO	36		30	TO	33		32	TO	35
32	TO	35		29	TO	32		31	TO	34
31	TO	34		28	TO	31		30	TO	33
30	TO	33		27	TO	30		29	TO	32
29	TO	32		26	TO	29		28	TO	31
28	TO	31		25	TO	28		27	TO	30
27	TO	30		24	TO	27		26	TO	29
26	TO	29		23	TO	26		25	TO	28
25	TO	28		22	TO	25		24	TO	27
24	TO	27		21	TO	24		23	TO	26

Hold ruler in a straight line across this chart. If clients measurements do not align straight across then move to the next chart and so on until you determine actual body shape.

TRIANGLE BODYSHAPE

BUST				WAIST				HIPS		
48	TO	51		53	TO	56		48	TO	51
47	TO	50		52	TO	55		47	TO	50
46	TO	49		51	TO	54		46	TO	49
45	TO	48		50	TO	53		45	TO	48
44	TO	47		49	TO	52		44	TO	47
43	TO	46		48	TO	51		43	TO	46
42	TO	45		47	TO	50		42	TO	45
41	TO	44		46	TO	49		41	TO	44
40	TO	43		45	TO	48		40	TO	43
39	TO	42		44	TO	47		39	TO	42
38	TO	41		43	TO	46		38	TO	41
37	TO	40		42	TO	45		37	TO	40
36	TO	39		41	TO	44		36	TO	39
35	TO	38		40	TO	43		35	TO	38
34	TO	37		39	TO	42		34	TO	37
33	TO	36		38	TO	41		33	TO	36
32	TO	35		37	TO	40		32	TO	35
31	TO	34		36	TO	39		31	TO	34
30	TO	33		35	TO	38		30	TO	33
29	TO	32		34	TO	37		29	TO	32
28	TO	31		33	TO	36		28	TO	31
27	TO	30		32	TO	35		27	TO	30
26	TO	29		31	TO	34		26	TO	29
25	TO	28		30	TO	33		25	TO	28
24	TO	27		29	TO	32		24	TO	27

Hold ruler in a straight line across this chart. If clients measurements do not align straight across then move to the next chart and so on until you determine actual body shape.

ROUND BODYSHAPE

BUST				WAIST				HIPS		
48	TO	51		53	TO	56		48	TO	51
47	TO	50		52	TO	55		47	TO	50
46	TO	49		51	TO	54		46	TO	49
45	TO	48		50	TO	53		45	TO	48
44	TO	47		49	TO	52		44	TO	47
43	TO	46		48	TO	51		43	TO	46
42	TO	45		47	TO	50		42	TO	45
41	TO	44		46	TO	49		41	TO	44
40	TO	43		45	TO	48		40	TO	43
39	TO	42		44	TO	47		39	TO	42
38	TO	41		43	TO	46		38	TO	41
37	TO	40		42	TO	45		37	TO	40
36	TO	39		41	TO	44		36	TO	39
35	TO	38		40	TO	43		35	TO	38
34	TO	37		39	TO	42		34	TO	37
33	TO	36		38	TO	41		33	TO	36
32	TO	35		37	TO	40		32	TO	35
31	TO	34		36	TO	39		31	TO	34
30	TO	33		35	TO	38		30	TO	33
29	TO	32		34	TO	37		29	TO	32
28	TO	31		33	TO	36		28	TO	31
27	TO	30		32	TO	35		27	TO	30
26	TO	29		31	TO	34		26	TO	29
25	TO	28		30	TO	33		25	TO	28
24	TO	27		29	TO	32		24	TO	27

Hold ruler in a straight line across this chart. If clients measurements do not align straight across then move to the next chart and so on until you determine actual body shape.

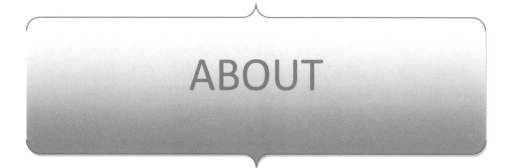

ABOUT

Gillian Armour Image Consulting Fact Sheet

Headquarters: Offices in Santa Fe, San Francisco and Honolulu

Telephone: Toll Free 1-800-591-2353

Web:

www.gillianarmour.com **(image tools, courses and seminars)**

www.albuquerquebootcamp.com **(fitness boot camps for women)**

www.armourgallery.com **(members only jewelry site)**

www.fashionimageinstitute.com **(online fashion, image and style e-courses)**

Since 2001, Gillian Armour Image Consulting, helmed by Gillian Armour, has helped men and women with their appearance, self-esteem, wardrobe, grooming and body language in ways that empower them to change.

Armour's background in fashion for companies like Macy's, I. Magnin and Jessica McClintock led her to open a full-service image consultancy to provide everything from simple makeovers to complex image overhauls as well as workshops and classes for clients and those who wish to pursue a career as an image consultant. Her studio includes a fashion library, hair and makeup areas, and a color and style analysis space.

Armour is the only Certified Image Professional in New Mexico and Hawaii, where she has a satellite office. She is certified by and a member of the Association of Image Consultants International (AICI). Clients include government, corporate and non-profit clients, as well as Fortune 500 Companies. Her extensive use of cutting edge technology allows her to consult in person and remotely, as well as teach classes and train image consultants in the U.S. and abroad from her headquarters.

While living in Hawaii, Armour began designing and creating her own line of jewelry, Gillian Armour Couture Jewels. Each one-of-a-kind piece features semi-precious stones sourced from green vendors who guarantee sustainable mining, harvesting and collection for the coral, pearls, turquoise and other gems in the line.

In 2006, Armour relocated from Hawaii to Santa Fe, and then to Albuquerque in 2007. The same year, she founded Albuquerque Adventure Boot Camp for Women, and is a certified Boot Camp Instructor. The daily exercise camps now serve the entire Albuquerque metropolitan area, having trained over 300 women in its first year.

Armour has published several books about fashion, color and body type, and has just completed a how-to guide to becoming an image consultant. In 2007, she formed Best Dressed^{sm} to help men, women and teens from economically challenged backgrounds enter the workforce by offering free of charge makeover and wardrobe services to qualified clients actively seeking employment. Best Dressed^{sm} is a 501(c) 3 nonprofit organization.

Associations and Certifications

- Certified Image Professional, Association of Image Consultants (AICI)
- Certified Lumina® Color Analysis Professional, Donna Fujii
- Certified Fashion Stylist and Personal Shopper, Fashion Image Institute(FII)
- Certified Personal Trainer, Circuit Training Instructor, Group Fitness and EZ8 Running, National Exercise & Sports Trainers Association (NESTA)
- Certified in Sports Nutrition, American Sport and Fitness Association (ASFA)
- Member National Speakers Association

WORKSHOPS

Recent training programs and workshops:

HOW TO GET THE MOST FROM YOUR EXISTING WARDROBE

Your budget tells you that you cannot afford another thing and besides your closet is already full of great clothes to wear. So what if some are last year's styles? Find out how you can update those styles. Learn to look at your existing clothing collection with newer, fresher eyes. Together we review the latest trends in fashion and show you how to match them with what you already may own. Discover how to tailor or change the cut of a jacket, pants or top to make it more relevant to today's styling.

- How to coordinate your clothes and have more to wear.
- How many ways can you wear a white shirt? Sound like a trick question? The answer is – as many ways as you can think of.
- Learn how to think about your wardrobe basics this way and how doing so will increase your options for what to wear.
- Together we plan with spreadsheets how you can take that white shirt and add color via accessories and jewelry to create a bigger, better selection.
- Workbook shows you how to coordinate by using the color wheel and color rules thereby increasing your menu of wearable choices.

BARGAIN AND BUDGET SHOPPING

Everybody knows that bargain shopping in department stores these days is like having the cherry on the cake – it's so easy to find sale items and bargains. But let's not overlook the smaller stores and the antique collectives. Even the big box retailers offer quality and stylish fashion at great prices. In this group class you will learn:

- How to think outside the box of your traditional shopping patterns to find chic, unique fashion choices.
- To plan for your purchases instead of just hunting for the latest, greatest and cheapest.
- What it takes to be fashion savvy and bargain happy when the choices are mind-boggling.

- How not to fall victim to fads and trends that cost you more (disposable fashion).
- To look for inexpensive (but quality) options for your working wardrobe.

MEND, SEW, TAILOR AND RE-FASHION YOUR WAY TO STYLE

Back in the day when we had money to burn most of us threw out or donated clothes that had rips, holes or stains. We wasted a lot of money and some really great fashion. It's time to be green about your clothing inventory. In this informative and fun class you will learn to:

- Edit and process the clothes in your closet that need TLC.
- Take another look at styles that no longer fit you and discover how to make them work.
- Create brand new styles from some of your old classics.
- Work with your tailor to shorten, lengthen, widen or shrink those clothes you have long sidelined.
- Let go the emotional hold you have on favorite styles that really no longer fit, flatter or shape you.

I NEVER DRY CLEAN – HOW I SAVED MYSELF $1250 IN ONE YEAR!

My mother was a great innovator and creative thinker. She had to come up with solutions to the enormous expenses of managing a family of ten people! I learned many cost-cutting methods from her especially when it came to taking care of clothes. We can all benefit from a mother's wisdom in this fashion boot camp class! You will discover how:

- To save a lot of money just by using the "hand wash" cycle of your washing machine.
- Discover why "Dry Clean Only" clothes are marked that way.
- Which fabrics really are "Dry Clean Only".
- Home dry cleaning kits – what they can and cannot do.
- What about difficult stains?

SHOW ME THE FASHION – CREATING A 15 PIECE WORKING WARDROBE FOR UNDER $500

Sound impossible? Not in my book. As a professional shopper it's my job to work within the budget limitations of my clients so I have learnt to shop at all levels of a fashion budget.

Find out that you don't have to limit your budget shopping to department and specialty shops and:

- Discover how to catalog shop, planning coordinates as you peruse your options.
- Discover how to hunt and pick from the sales racks for "bang for buck" merchandise.
- Plan a 15 piece wardrobe graph to mix-n-match and extend your wearable choices.
- Choose accessories that upgrade, embellish and extend plain looks.
- Put your personal spin on classic sportswear and look like a million.

DIY – HAIR, NAILS AND FACIALS AND SAVE $$$

Here's a challenge for you fashionistas out there – make a list of how much you spend every month on pedicures, manicures, haircuts, colors and facials. That's the money you could save by doing-it-yourself (DIY). As they say "a penny saved is a penny earned" so what better way to save a few than to learn how to pamper yourself? During this class you will discover:

- How to find great prices on beauty services and supplies.
- Discount salons – the good, the bad and the one's to avoid.
- Beauty Schools – how to pick and choose from their menu's.
- Gratis products and samples – learn how to ask for these freebies.
- Where to get your makeup done – for FREE.

YOUR CLOSET IS FULL OF SURPRISES – 10 WAYS TO GET MORE STYLE FROM EXISTING CLOTHING PIECES

Do you find yourself in a clothing rut with nothing exciting to wear? Do you tend to wear the same favorite pieces over and over again rarely mixing it up? There is good news – discover the surprises your closet will yield AFTER you have emptied it completely. This fun workshop introduces you to the idea of radical change and re-invention plus:

- How purging your closet leads to re-inventing a whole new wardrobe.
- Find long lost favorites in your closet and put them to good use.
- Get rid of the un-wearables, the un-bearables and the un-desireables.
- Plan a dress-up day with best friends and re-discover what you love about your clothes.
- How throwing a "Girlfriend's Closet Party" will release your attachment to old clothes.

THE IMPORTANCE OF FEELING GOOD IN YOUR CLOTHES

Do the clothes you wear make you feel frumpy and dumpy or confident and beautiful? Is the way you dress telling the world who you really are? Do you dress to impress others and forsake how you feel in your own clothes?

- Discover your "style personality" and how it reveals itself through your clothing and accessory choices.
- Take the Style Personality Quiz and get the answers to looking and feeling better.
- Discover a style that is uniquely you, that gives you a greater sense of self.
- Explore options for dressing to a changing body.
- Make impressions about you that count.

IMAGE SERVICES

Research has shown that a poor image can be professionally costly as well as personally painful. Both individuals and companies can experience tremendous benefits by improving their image. That's why a growing number of people are turning to professional image consultants.

"Today, image professionals are beginning to be on the same level as Interior designers. Anyone who wants to look their best and be appropriate will now hire an image consultant." Anna Soo Wildermuth, AICI President.

As a professional *and* certified international image consultant, I specialize in visual appearance and non-verbal communication. I counsel individual and corporate clients on appearance, behavior, and communication skills through individual consultations, coaching, presentations, seminars and workshops. My Image Consultancy is not about a radical makeover or plastic surgery; it is about helping you with your appearance, wardrobe, grooming, and body language in a way that empowers you to change.

My company, Gillian Armour Image Consulting, is allied with other trained and certified experts from image related fields. Together we work with you to custom tailor a complete image package for all your appearance needs. From a simple makeover to complex visual branding consultations, the following is a list of services we offer that are geared toward helping you achieve your maximum potential as a well dressed person.

- Image in Business
- Visual Branding
- Image Analysis
- Image for Men
- Body/Shape Analysis
- On Line Analysis Programs
- Wardrobe Edit/ Closet Organizing
- Custom Color Analysis
- Makeup Consultation
- Etiquette Skills Training
- Non-Verbal Communication Consultation
- Personal Shopping
- Personal Style interview

- Appearance Evaluation
- Body Shape, Fit and Sizing
- Evaluation of Non-Verbal Communication
- Evaluation of Communication Skills
- Style Collage and Core Wardrobe Workbook
- Shopping Preferences and Plans
- What is Image?
- What Does it Take to be Successful?
- Basic Professional Wardrobe Capsule
- Purchase Planning
- Sample Wardrobe with Pictures (5 outfits on mannequin)
- Wardrobe Hints
- Wardrobe Planning
- Investment Dressing
- Image Checklist
- Fabric Information
- Eyewear Guide
- The Job Interview
- Dating Attire Do's and Don'ts
- Head shot/Portrait Planning
- Fashion Styling

BOOKS BY GILLIAN ARMOUR

- Mastering the Art of Dressing Well
- Mastering the Art of Business Image
- Mastering the Art of Image Consulting
- Glamour Girls Guide to Looking Gorgeous
- How to Dress Guide - Asian Body
- Reigning Over Closet Chaos
- Are You Coordinated?
- Ten Steps to Absolute Chic
- How to Do an Image Consult
- Social Media Marketing for Image Consultants
- How to Write and Produce and E-Book
- What's Your Style Personality?

PRODUCTS @ www.gillianarmour.com

- Color Season Makeup
- Custom Color Analysis
- Color Season Guides
- Body Shape Guides
- Royalty Free jpeg's for Fashion Coordination
- Licensing program "My Style Firm" for certified fashion stylists and image consultants
- E-Books
- E-Courses

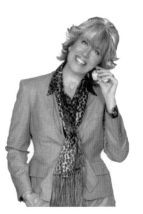

Gillian Armour, AICI CIP,

Image Consultant /Celebrity Stylist and the fashion columnist for Albuquerque's *Sage Magazine*. Gillian appeared for several seasons on the award winning NBC show *"Dream Makeover Hawaii"* as its official image consultant and stylist.

As a Style Director Gillian has produced fashion shows, photography shoots, TV commercials and TV Movies. She has styled many celebrities and teaches a certified course for budding Fashion Stylists.

Her career in retail fashion reaches back 25 years and includes executive, managerial and buying positions with retailers *Macy's, I. Magnin* and *House of Fraser*, London.

Gillian is the author of many eBooks on image and writes for successful fashion social networking sites. Gillian was recently named a Beauty Expert for several high fashion magazines and blogs about fashion, style and image frequently.

NOTES

NOTES

Made in the USA
Charleston, SC
19 April 2010